VEGUCATION
OVER
MEDICATION

The Myths, Lies, and Truths About Modern Foods and Medicines

DR. BOBBY PRICE

Plant-Based Pharmacist; Fitness & Nutrition Expert

healing. Each person's health needs are unique and often require individual attention. To address your specific needs, please consult your personal healthcare provider.

Copyright 2018 Bobby J. Price, Pharm.D.

Printed in the United States of America

Published by Wise Old Owl Publishing

International Standard Book Number: 978-0-9996124-0-8

Contents

About the Author

D r. Bobby J. Price is a certified plant-based nutritionist, exercise physiologist and Doctor of Pharmacy. He has extensive clinical experience in the hospital setting, one-on-one patient contact in community pharmacy, and health care regulatory experience with the Food and Drug Administration (FDA).

After personally experiencing the healing powers of a plant-based lifestyle seven years ago, he was inspired to adopt a more holistic approach to healing others. Since that time, he has traveled the world studying with herbalists, shamans, and spiritual gurus, learning the magical arts of healing the mind, body, and soul. Now, instead of filling synthetic prescriptions, he uses plant-based foods, medicinal herbs, and simple holistic techniques to help others restore their well-being.

In *Vegucation Over Medication,* he exposes the myths, lies, and truths about modern foods and medicines. He believes that when aligned with nature, our bodies have an innate ability to heal and the responsibility of our health can be placed back into our hands— where it belongs.

You can find Dr. Price on Facebook, Twitter, and Instagram.

1.

Vegucation Over Medication

Let Food Be Your Medicine, Medicine Be Your Food.
—Imhotep, 2600 BCE

I n 2011, I was eating a lion's share of meat daily and handing out medications like lifesavers to drowning victims. I truly believed my work as a pharmacist was saving lives and making a difference in my community.

I had started my career in healthcare with the audacity to believe that modern medicine could stop disease and, in some cases, even cure patients. In pharmacy school, we had learned all about the new cutting-edge technologies and upcoming advances in medicine. We all believed that one day, illness would be a thing of the past.

I've always felt most fulfilled when I was caring for someone. It wasn't uncommon for me to pay for a patient's prescription when it was too expensive and even go to a patient's house to explain how to use an insulin pen or glucose meter. Over time, I began to understand that something wasn't right. That protective layer of a sense of fulfillment started to wither away. Despite the best efforts of our healthcare system, every day it seemed like I was seeing a new patient who had been handed a life sentence to high blood pressure, diabetes, an autoimmune disorder, or cancer.

Even with all the advances in technology and medicine, it's more common for people to be sick than healthy in America. Our drinking water is contaminated, the air is polluted, foods are tainted with chemicals, and medical errors are the third leading cause of death after heart disease and cancer. I was beginning to feel less and less like a *healer* and more like a *dealer*.

Even I was not immune to chronic disease. Since the age of sixteen, despite being an athlete with less than 8% body fat, I had been struggling with hypertension. Like most people, I figured it was hereditary, and there was nothing I could do about it. As a result, during every doctor's visit, I would receive a prescription and ultimately refuse to take it. This should come as no surprise because most healthcare practitioners make the worst patients, and I wasn't

an exception. The concept "once you have it, you got it" was

ingrained in my psyche during pharmacy school. To my knowledge,

chronic diseases could only be managed, not cured.

It wasn't until I decided to adopt a plant-based vegan

lifestyle for 60 days as a means to lose my belly fat that the idea of

heredity as a health predetermination began to come unraveled. I

was only hoping to lose maybe ten pounds at best during the

challenge, and I was pretty skeptical about that. But instead, I lost 35

pounds and six inches off my waistline and eased the aches and

pains in my joints. The tingling sensations in my legs ceased, my

keg turned into a six-pack, and the elevated blood pressure I had

since a teen normalized. My blood pressure dropped from a typical

average of 160/95 to 120/74. I couldn't believe it!

I ended up getting several colleagues to recheck my pressure

just to confirm that I had, in fact, been cured. I instantly became an

evangelist at the counseling window, especially for patients with

high blood pressure, giving them my personal testimony. Everyone

was asking me what I had done to lose the weight because it was

such a dramatic shift in such a short amount of time. I explained how my plant-based prescription that included green juices and smoothies had healed me. I shared my recipes and told them the foods they needed to restrict.

One by one, they came back to share their own success stories. What was even more shocking was discovering they weren't just being cured of high blood pressure but almost every condition for which they were being treated. Patients who suffered from diabetes for decades balanced their blood sugars. The weight melted off their waistlines like butter. Cholesterol levels plummeted. Joint inflammation disappeared. Hormonal imbalances were restored, and they experienced increased energy with glowing skin tones and pain-free menses, just to name a few positive side effects.

Before I knew it, patients were showing up at my counseling window, asking me for 'the cure' in a whisper. Sometimes patients would call and ask what they had to do to get better, so I would begin to give them conventional medical advice. They would quickly interrupt and say, "Not that way, doc. Your natural way! Maybe I should have come into the pharmacy instead of calling?"

They were speaking as if I were doing something illegal! This made me realize that while what I was doing wasn't illegal, it wasn't good for business. In our current healthcare system, it's frowned upon to replace medical advice with a holistic approach. I can remember working for the Food and Drug Administration (FDA), fielding calls from patients who had been injured by prescriptions and attending drug approval hearings, thinking that our design for healing was flawed and, in many cases, bordering criminal mischief.

And only a few years later, I had become an instrument for that system in a community pharmacy!

I decided right there I wanted better for patients and better for myself. I realized that what my friends, colleagues, and patients needed was not *medication* but *vegucation*. They needed to understand and embrace a new approach to the food they ate and embark on a new journey towards good health.

Then the opportunity came for me to leave the United States and move to Okinawa, Japan, where I was able to study one of the healthiest populations of Centenarians (people who live to be one hundred or more years old) in the world. With my newfound knowledge of what a healthy lifestyle looked like, I leaped at the chance. I was especially excited because, in an effort to understand why so many younger patients were getting ill and dying so early, I had started researching Centenarians around the world. When the offer came in 2013, I realized I had been studying the same people living 11,000 miles away whom I would soon be meeting!

The Centenarians of Okinawa

Despite being a small and densely populated island, Okinawa has consistently had one of the highest proportions of centenarians in the world. I lived on the island for more than three years, routinely visiting a small village named Ogimi, home to more than a dozen centenarians. Each time, I was shocked to see people in their nineties, and even over one hundred years old, riding bikes, walking up hilly terrains, farming and enthralled in joyful conversation with each other. What was even more impressive was the quality of life they enjoyed at the century mark. Many were disease-free, with minds sharp as tacks, and still physically capable of manual labor.

It was common for me, as a healthcare practitioner, to see someone in their forties riddled with disease and with a quality of life that was just above a death certificate. In stark contrast to the Standard American Diet (which carries the ironic acronym of SAD), these Okinawans consumed an array of seasonal vegetables and fruits that were organic, anti-inflammatory, nutritionally dense and contained phytonutrients capable of stomping out cancer. Instead of the fried syrupy breakfast we prefer in the United States, herbal teas and sea vegetables constituted a typical morning meal for them.

During my time in Okinawa, I would ask local friends to take me to Ogimi Village to visit either their grandparents or friends of their family who were still spry at the age of 100 years or more. They would talk to me about their lifestyle and allow me to be a witness to it. Walking through their gardens was like going into an armory of weapons for good health. The foods they grew were an arsenal against virtually every disease known to man and a perfect protocol for longevity.

Their staple vegetable was the nutrient-packed *Beni-imo* (purple sweet potato), which represented over two-thirds of their vegetable consumption. It's high in vitamins A and C and manganese but also helps regulate blood sugar while demonstrating an antifungal and anti-bacterial effect. There were vegetables like *Goya* (bitter melon) that also helps to balance blood sugar and reduce HbA1c (shorthand for hemoglobin A1C or glycosylated

hemoglobin) for diabetic patients.

They also grew mugwort ,luffa, fruit and turmeric. Mugwort

is anti-epileptic, stimulates gastric juices and bile secretions during

digestion, helps regulate menstruation and can aid in depression.

Then there was the *luffa* fruit (*luffa* gourd), which is extremely high

in vitamins, minerals, and antioxidants. It also treats colds and sinus

infections and can be dehydrated and used as a sponge. Turmeric

root, which is naturally anti-inflammatory, has been clinically

proven to prevent and fight cancer and lowers the risk of heart

disease. They ate *mozuku*, which is a form of seaweed rich in

vitamin K that improves blood circulation, reduces cholesterol, and

boosts the immune system.

These were just a few of the foods they grew and ate on a

daily basis. I also saw pineapples, oranges with green skins and

heavily seeded, and green papaya growing in the wild. Just as

Imhotep had advised over four thousand years ago, these people

were literally making food their medicine and medicine their food.

I was able to use the military libraries on the bases in

Okinawa, where they kept extensive records of the Okinawans' diets and lifestyles both prior to and after the American war with Japan. The U.S. National Archives kept food records in 1949 based on a survey of 2,279 persons done after WWII before the U.S. turned Okinawa back over to Japan. I discovered that Okinawans did, in fact, eat very small portions of meat, most often as small cubes of pork used for flavoring vegetables. They sparingly ate fish, usually a portion size less than half the palm of their hands. All in all, meat and dairy represented only 3% of their diet.

The remainder of the Okinawan diet overwhelmingly consisted of plant-based foods, with a very small percentage of processed foods. It was also interesting to discover that because the foods they ate were so nutritionally dense, they only ate about 1,800 calories per day; however, by weight, they ate significantly more than a typical meat eater would. This type of diet is high in fiber and antioxidants and is highly anti-inflammatory.

According to a 2010 article in *Current Gerontology and Geriatrics Research*, the diet of Okinawan was laden with antioxidants, making their free radical levels significantly lower by more than 50%. This heavily reduces their risk for cancer. This study also determined this was not based on genetics; their antioxidant activity was the same as individuals who lived into their eighties, and it was the excess antioxidants consumed in their plant-based diets that afforded them the additional health.

This is a reflection of the culture, as it is common for mothers, grandmothers, and physicians to use the old phrase "Hara Hachi Bu" (*Hara* means stomach, *Hachi* is the number 8, and *Bu* means level). This statement translates to: "Don't eat until you are full (10), stop at 8." However, the caloric restriction of their diet does not supersede the plant-based nature of it. When compared to the Loma Linda California Adventists, vegetarians have the highest life expectancy of any formally described population and eat a 100% meatless diet. These particular Adventist vegetarians have an average life expectancy of 83.3 and 85.7 years for men and women respectively. These averages were slightly better compared to Okinawan men, whose average age was 77.6 years in 2000, and comparable to Okinawan women who averaged 86 years.

The best group among them was the Adventist vegetarians, who incorporated healthy lifestyles as well, such as not smoking and consistent exercise. The life expectancy for men was 87 and women was 89.6 years on average.

Their diet and lifestyle explains why Okinawans experience up to three times fewer deaths from colon cancer, are 5.5 times less likely to die from breast cancer, seven times less likely to die from prostate cancer, and up to a 12-fold reduction in death from heart disease.

I spoke in detail with many of the elders in the village and learned a lot about the myths and misperceptions we have around food in America. Even the idea that Japanese are leaner and healthier as a result of genetics and a faster metabolism is based on myth. The elder explained that because of the remote location of Ogimi in the north of the island, the locals maintained their traditions of eating and living, uninfluenced by the poor eating habits of westerners located in the central part of the island. After World War II, the U.S. military occupied this tiny island for 27 years, up until 1972. Although the U.S. relinquished control of Okinawa almost 45 years ago, many of their family members who had moved to the central parts of the islands adopted the American tradition of fast food. For the first time, the elders saw disease and obesity in their families.

Probably one of the most dangerous collateral side effects of the American invasion was the introduction of burgers and fries with A&W fast food chains, Spam luncheon meat made popular by young soldiers, and now more than a dozen KFCs on the island. Case by case, the villagers gave me countless stories about slender granddaughters who had married American soldiers and left Okinawa to move to the States, only to return overweight. They spoke of sons and nephews who had moved near American bases and had fallen in love with the foods that catered to the military began to experience obesity and heart disease.

The longevity that Okinawans once possessed is now becoming a thing of the past. Upon my arrival in 2013, the tiny island was already riddled with fast-food restaurants. Despite being in possession of the secret sauce to longevity, the locals have embraced a Western diet, and in just two generations, Okinawans have transitioned from being the leanest group in Japan to now among the fattest.

This makes it clear that the argument of genetics is not the deciding factor in health determination. But it doesn't explain what is it about eating meat that leads to poor health. The Western-style diet, more popularly known as SAD diet, is composed of 25% meat and its by-products, 63% processed foods, and 12% plant foods. Some form of white potato is 50% of the 12% of plant foods eaten in the form of mashed potatoes, French fries, or baked potato.

In contrast, the traditional Okinawan diet was composed of just 1% meat and its by-products. That was true vegucation!

Studying in India

When I moved to India to learn yoga, meditation, and Ayurvedic medicine, my perspective on the human body completely evolved. I honestly don't know if before coming to India I had a perspective beyond anatomy, biology, and reproduction of the body. In India, I learned our body is the temple for our soul. It's how we experience the external world through our sensory perceptions, while the mind is how we experience our internal environment where the soul resides.

Instead of looking at ourselves as people here only to work, reproduce, and die, we are spiritual beings here to have a human experience, not vice versa. Our bodies and minds are our tools to have this experience.

With this perspective, it would then make sense for us to have the best possible experience. We should maintain our vehicle of life in top shape to better enhance our perceptions and have the highest experience possible.

Practicing yoga and meditation at the K. Pattabhi Jois Ashtanga Yoga Institute in Mysore, India, helped me to create a beautiful union between my mind and body. The practice has a spiritual focus that is guided by the breath and moved by the body. The poses are masterfully organized in sequential order to cleanse, heal, and restore the body back to its factory settings. While the chanting and meditation help to re-establish a peaceful mental balance that calms the nervous system, alleviates stress and reduces the heart rate and blood pressure.

I also learned that Ayurvedic medicine, much like traditional Indian cuisine, used food as medicine. Like the Okinawans, the foods recommended for yogis was Ayurvedic cooking that contained medicinal herbs like turmeric, cumin, ginger, fenugreek, coriander, cardamom amongst others that heal the body.

The Amazing Human Body

This vehicle, the human body, is by far the most complicated piece of machinery in existence on Earth. Here are a few amazing facts about the magnificent machinery you possess:

- The stomach's digestive acids are strong enough to not only digest zinc but the tissues around it. However, the cells lining the stomach regenerate at such a rapid rate it makes it impossible to dissolve them.

- The brain produces the electrical energy equivalent to a 20-watt light bulb, which would explain the comparison of a lit light bulb over our heads when we have a great epiphany.

- You would need 82,000 processors for a supercomputer to simulate just one second of 1% of our brain's capacity.

- Ounce for ounce, human bone is stronger than granite or steel, yet it weighs three times less. One cubic inch of human bone (about the size of a matchbox) is capable of supporting the weight of five pickup trucks, or roughly nine tons—this is four times as much as concrete. The engineering of human bone is so magnificently efficient and strong it has become a template for many modern engineering projects, including buildings and bridges.

- A man's testicles can manufacture up to 10 million sperm cells daily. Which makes a man capable of repopulating the entire planet in six months.

- The human body is made of seven octillion atoms. As a comparison, our entire galaxy is made of only 300 billion stars.

- Ninety percent of our cells aren't even human in origin! Most are fungi and bacteria.

- The skin is replaced every two weeks.

- Every 120 days, our entire blood supply is replaced.

- Every 300 days, through the brilliance of our divine engineering, we have a new liver.

- Every ten years, we get an entirely new skeletal system.

The Key to Health Is Plant-Based Food

All of this wizardry doesn't happen with a hidden magic wand.

The magic is in our food. The foods we eat are used to recreate that which took nine months to manifest in our mother's womb and 18 or more years to mature in the physical world. So the body you so greatly identify with is a very fluid concept, and you are much younger than you think. However, if you eat fast and cheap foods, you will age quickly and deteriorate at the same pace. But if you adopt a plant-based diet lifestyle, devoid of meat, dairy, and processed pseudo-foods, you'll maintain a youthful appearance, live a higher quality of life with less disease and have the opportunity to die peacefully in your sleep at 100 plus years old.

As complicated as this machinery may seem, the primary building block of your physical body is simply your nutrition. You literally are what you eat. But just like any other highly sophisticated machinery, our bodies have specific guidelines and manufacturer's requirements for optimal use. Like gas for cars, our fuel (food) should be of the highest quality and packed with energy to give us the vitality that defines life and not a zombie-like state of living.

Too Many Americans Are Sick

America boasts the most expensive and technologically advanced healthcare system in the world, yet it's not designed to *keep people healthy*, only to *treat them when they're sick*. Our healthcare system actually has no place for a healthy person!

The truth is, in America, we don't have healthcare; what we have is *sick care*.

One of the biggest reasons is because there's no money in treating either deceased people or healthy patients. The money to be made is right in the middle, from those individuals teetering on the line between life and death riddled with chronic diseases, each organ system failing slowly and one at a time. If it's the pancreas, we call it diabetes; if it's the heart, we call it cardiovascular disease, and so on. The majority of drugs are designed to manipulate our biochemistry just enough to prolong life and create a lifelong customer.

I'm not insinuating that your doctor wants you to be ill. In actuality, I believe that out of love, most doctors make an enormous sacrifice of their health to undertake the grueling task of becoming a physician to care for others. Unfortunately, most healthcare professionals are educated by the same system that by and large is funded and educated by Big Pharma. So we are just as frustrated with not being able to cure you as you are with not being cured.

The greatest whoppers to the health care of Americans (pun intended) are heart disease and stroke. At a price tag of $432 billion annually, cardiovascular disease is responsible for one in every four deaths in America. This will probably come as no surprise, considering most people know that cardiovascular disease is the number one cause of death for both men and women in the United States.

However, what may shock you and your physician is the knowledge that the number one cause of premature death in the U.S. is directly related to the SAD diet, not heredity. What we inherit are the eating habits of our family. And yet it seems that whenever there is scientific and clinical discussion around a solution for chronic diseases, nutrition is the invisible 800-pound gorilla in the room. Modern medicine can't be the answer because there's never been so much medical spending, yet Americans are getting sicker and dying earlier in epidemic numbers.

This is precisely why despite being a pharmacist, I advocate for *Vegucation Over Medication*. I'm not entirely against medication because, in acute situations, drugs have lifesaving capabilities. I also understand that people have a right to choose what they eat, and so medications become necessary to manipulate our body's biochemistry. But most people are either misinformed or uninformed about which can foods heal, as opposed to those that kill. The purpose of this book is to educate and explain how many of your comfort foods cause illness, and plant-based lifestyle is the greatest form of prevention and disease reversal.

Food Can Be Medicine

The use of food as medicine has a long recorded history that spans thousands of years, even before the time of Hippocrates, and today it still remains at the center of healing disease. Did you know that up to 50% of all recently approved drugs worldwide have a plant-based origin, either directly or indirectly? Many of you are enjoying the therapeutic benefits of these drugs every day without knowing.

- The ancient Egyptians used willow bark for the same aches and pains as you do—but you probably know it as aspirin.
- The drug digoxin used to treat heart arrhythmias is derived from the plant *Digitalis Purpurea*.
- Etoposide, an anti-tumor agent, used in the treatment of cancer, is derived from the mayapple plant.

This list could literally wrap around a building, but what's important to understand is, although these drugs are derived from plants, they are very different from their natural parents. The pharmaceutical drugs are filled with chemicals, dyes, and fillers that end up creating the long list of potential side effects you experience. If you consumed it as a whole food instead, you would not only receive the medicinal benefits but also the nutritional and cleansing effect.

We as healthcare professionals should be vegucating our patients on the miracles of a whole-foods, plant-based lifestyle as our primary form of prevention and disease reversal. But instead, we passively mention the importance of diet and aggressively prescribe drugs.

Warfarin: From Rat Poison to Blood Thinner

Patients who are dehydrated and are eating sugary and fatty foods can cause their blood to become viscous, reducing circulation. This also increases the potential for blood cells to stick together and form clots. These clots can form in the leg and cause deep vein thrombosis or dislodge and go to the heart to cause a heart attack or to the brain, leading to a fatal stroke.

Such patients are typically placed on a blood thinner called Coumadin.

Here's where the plot thickens. The active ingredient, warfarin, was initially formulated as a *rat poison*, and it acted by thinning the rodents' blood so much they died from massive internal bleeding. Since 1954, it has been prescribed to humans as a blood thinner! The risk for bleeding is so high that it requires the patient's clotting factors be constantly monitored in order to ensure the patient is properly dosed.

As Aureolus Paracelsus (1493–1541), the 'Grandfather of Pharmacology,' wrote, "All things are poisons, for there is nothing without poisonous qualities. It is only the dose which makes a thing a poison. A lot kills, a little cures." In the case of Warfarin: short term, it can be life-saving, but long-term, the continued poor habits along with the side effects of the drug can potentially be fatal.

I once had a patient who had lived in Argentina for a number of years learning to become a tango dancer. Because of my love for traveling, we spent much time talking at the counseling window about his experiences living abroad. He was an older gentleman with enough youthful vigor to still dance the night away, and I was a young pharmacist inspired by his experiences. One day while in mid-conversation, I noticed his nose started bleeding. I quickly grabbed a tissue and sat him down. I knew that he had been taking Warfarin for years, and it was a few days after Thanksgiving, so the first question I asked was if he had eaten an unusual amount of green leafy vegetables during his Thanksgiving feasting.

He explained that in an attempt to eat a more plant-based diet, he had eaten several plates of his mother's tasty collard greens.

The irony is that the first counseling point we are trained to educate patients taking warfarin is: "Continue to eat your typical portion size of green vegetables." This is because green leafy vegetables contain vitamin K, which helps to clot the blood and makes Warfarin ineffective. Many patients start avoiding green vegetables all together at this point, but that's where we allow our decisions to be influenced by myths. It is not necessary for you to avoid eating greens. The cause for concern is with dramatic shifts in the amount of greens you consume while taking a blood thinner. However, it's important to decide on a set amount daily and then speak with your doctor so that it can be built into your therapy and the drug dosage can be adjusted. Eventually, with continued effort, your blood will become naturally thin, and your physician can wean you off Warfarin.

As I mentioned before, pharmaceutical drugs can be life-saving in acute situations such as embolic stroke or if a patient has a mechanical heart valve. But over the long-term, it's imperative to transition to a more holistic alternative because artificially thinning the blood instead of addressing the cause of clotting will eventually catch up with you.

Eating large amounts of animal protein, eggs, dairy, and processed foods causes the blood to be viscous and concentrated. When blood is stagnant and dehydrated, it sets the stage for blood cells to aggregate together and leads to clots. Plant-based foods are loaded with hydration and nutrients that naturally thin the blood while also providing vitamin K2 to produce clots, which are necessary if you happen to cut yourself.

What You Don't Know About Statin Drugs

Here's another case where vegucation is more necessary than medication. If you look up the connection between cholesterol and its impact on cardiovascular health, you'll get a ton of conflicting information from both credible and layman sources. But what can't be disputed is the fact that Lipitor, a cholesterol-lowering drug, in a class of drugs known as statins, is the best-selling drug of all time. What shouldn't be confused is the phrase 'best-selling' with 'most effective,' because the rate of cardiovascular deaths is still the leading cause of death globally to the tune of 17.7 million lives annually. Coronary artery disease, the narrowing of arteries caused by fatty plaques, is responsible for 850,000 opportunities annually for surgeons to crack open the chests of Americans to surgically implant stents. These surgeons have a first-hand view of the impact of meat, dairy, and processed vegetable oils on our vascular health due to inflammation and fatty deposits.

What needs to be understood is that the words 'fat' and 'cholesterol' are not synonymous.

Cholesterol gets a bad reputation because only the tragic side of its story is told. In fact, cholesterol is present in the membranes of every cell in our body. It's essential for making vital hormones like vitamin D, testosterone, and estrogen, and in the production of bile acids, which are responsible for dissolving digested fats. Eighty percent of our cholesterol is made by the liver and intestines at night while we're comfortably asleep. We only require 20% of our cholesterol from dietary sources.

Health becomes disease when we over-consume processed fats, sugars, and unhealthy proteins that are later converted into triglycerides and the type of cholesterol that clogs arteries. For instance, if you have two eggs every morning for breakfast (each containing 200 mg of cholesterol), the liver will, in turn, produce 1,600 mg of cholesterol. According to the Mayo Clinic, healthy individuals should consume no more than 300 mg of cholesterol daily. You can easily see how quickly your cholesterol levels could explode, considering you ate just two eggs, not even including the bacon or pancakes saturated with syrup!

For the majority of patients, when their blood cholesterol levels begin to peak beyond 200 mg/dL, despite the risk of dangerous side effects, their physician will immediately put them on a statin drug. It is well known that statins can deplete your body of the enzyme CoQ10, which is directly involved in energy production in the cells. This is what produces the side effect of fatigue that's often experienced. Statins can also cause memory loss, increased risk for diabetes, liver damage, muscle pain, and a life-threatening condition called rhabdomyolysis.

The truth is, while statins can be very effective at lowering your blood cholesterol levels, new studies are showing that this does not correlate to a reduction in cardiovascular disease and could be putting you at an increased risk for a cardiovascular incident. According to a 2015 report published in the *Expert Review for Clinical Pharmacology*, the initial clinical studies that validated the efficacy of statins used a statistical manipulation tool called Relative Risk Reduction (RRR) to exaggerate the mediocre benefits of the drugs. When compared with the absolute risk, it was discovered that these drugs are only effective for 1% of the entire population (1 out of 100 persons).

My father had a first-hand encounter with statins. While I was living in Japan, he suffered a stroke, and unbeknownst to me, his physician prescribed him Atorvastatin 40mg (Lipitor). Months later, my father began to complain of being lethargic and forgetful. This was especially odd because my father was always able to recall detailed memories from my childhood even I wasn't able to remember. When I asked if he was still walking the neighborhood for exercise, he said he wasn't able to walk forty yards away from the house because he would get tired and have extreme leg pain. In addition, his blood sugar began to spin out of control.

It's very common in health care to misinterpret drug side effects as signs of aging, and this is exactly what was happening to my father.

After informing his physician and discontinuing the drug, within six months, the symptoms had begun to resolve themselves.

This is another case where addressing the *symptoms* instead of the *cause* can lead to more harm than good. If we as healthcare professionals were equally as aggressive with counseling patients on necessary lifestyle adjustments as we are with handing out prescriptions, then the vast majority of drug therapy would become obsolete. Had my father been properly educated about what foods were causing the elevated cholesterol levels and which plant-based sources to use as replacements, he would have never had to suffer from the ill effects of statin drugs or subsequently have had his gallbladder removed.

Healthcare Professionals and Patients Need to Be Vegucated

In my opinion, it would be unfair to place all the blame in the lap of the physician. After all, at the vast majority of medical schools, students are not required to take even a single course on the subject of nutrition, and it's only offered at 25% of schools as an elective. Asking the average physician about nutrition would be the equivalent of asking a policeman to defend you in a court of law. Our common sense tells us that in each case, the subject matter is related to the professional, but in both cases, they are most often ill-prepared to be of any service. The belief that we can eat whatever we want and then use a 'magic pill' as to fix any problems is precisely why 70% of all Americans are taking at least one prescription. The bulk of modern foods we've developed an emotional connection to have addiction engineered into the ingredients. The foods we think we love so desperately are just a false representation of the nourishing relationship we could be having with plant-based whole foods. Instead, we're in this toxic relationship with processed foods and drugs.

For over a century, the astronomical cost of health has been rising directly in correlation with disease. That blatantly says that despite the fact we have the best medical technology and spend more health care dollars than any other country in the world, the system is failing.

More importantly, it tells us *you cannot buy good health.*

2.

The Cause of Disease:

Toxic Overload

If prevention can be accomplished, then cures will not be needed. –Dr. J.H. Tilden

S ince 1938, over 1,453 drugs have gained FDA approval all in the name of curing people of their various illnesses. Yet not one of these drugs has even cured the simplest ailment, the common cold.

The failures of modern medicine are due largely in part to its *reductionist approach* to healing the human body. The reductionist philosophy believes that by addressing the part of the whole that is experiencing the greatest effect (symptom), a treatment can be developed. This 'divide and conquer' approach directly impacts how we diagnose and treat disease. Most of the science of diagnosis comes from studying disease either in dead bodies or on Petri dishes. This is why I say we don't have a *health care* system; what we have is *sick care*. It's only designed to treat the sick and dying. While healthy individuals are sent home until they can join the party.

We take this same approach when it comes to vitamin and mineral deficiencies. The doctor will attempt to treat individual deficiencies with corresponding vitamins and minerals. The majority of nutritional supplements are synthetic, but in nature, nutrients are provided in perfect divine ratios to each other, not in single servings.

We often see failures of this philosophy with patients. If a patient is anemic as a result of vitamin B12 deficiency but is misdiagnosed and then given folic acid as treatment, the laboratory results will show increased blood cell formation, and you will appear to be cured. Meanwhile, the vitamin B12 deficiency goes unnoticed; it can lead to nerve degeneration and potentially paralysis. Both vitamin B12 and folate are part of the B-complex vitamins, which can be found in plant-based whole foods to act as a form of prevention and remedy to this patient. The healthcare system approach to healing rarely addresses the *underlying cause*, so by default, it can never cure the disease. Cures only become necessary when we fail to take the proper prevention. But then again, prevention is only possible when you know the cause.

So let's get to the root cause.

The use of whole foods to cure disease isn't some new age trendy concept; it's a return to the original standard. From as far back as ancient Egypt, there are 3,000-year-old medical texts that document the use of plant-based foods to heal the same ailments we suffer from today. And just like modern humans, subsequent societies embraced advancement over nature, and their well-being suffered as a result.

The Power of Natural Vitamin C

There have been many fortuitous discoveries in establishing the connection between disease and nutrition, such as in 1497, when Vasco de Gama's crew discovered that "when life gives you scurvy, make lemonade." This was at a time when scurvy was the leading killer of men who took to the seas, and citrus fruits became their savior.

Now we know the active ingredient in citrus fruits that cured scurvy was natural vitamin C.

Did you know that most vitamins made today, whether they are fortified into cereals or encapsulated in supplements, are created in a laboratory? These synthetic versions are structurally identical to the vitamins present in whole foods, but their activity in the body is not. Even vitamins that are labeled 'natural' only require that 10% originate from plant-based foods. The other 90% is left up to the supplement manufacturer's discretion. With the exception of monkeys, guinea pigs, and humans, most animals are capable of making their own endogenous vitamin C by making a few alterations to glucose. Humans, unfortunately, don't synthesize certain enzymes, so we're required to get vitamin C from dietary sources.

Virtually all vitamin C sold today is in the form of ascorbic acid. Here's a rude awakening: *Ascorbic acid is not vitamin C.* It is an extracted isolate of vitamin C most often made with genetically modified high fructose corn syrup and other harsh chemicals. Vitamin C is a complex that includes ascorbinogen, bioflavonoids, factors (J, K, P), rutin, and tyrosinase. Vitamin C also requires mineral co-factors in proper ratios. If any of these supporting factors are absent, then there will be no biological activity. The benefits of vitamin C—including immune boosting, wound healing, collagen formation, iron absorption, and tissue repairing—can only be received when we consume it in its whole form from plant-based foods. This was confirmed in 1937 by Nobel Prize Laureate Dr. Albert Szent-Georgi, who discovered the chemical structure for vitamin C. The conclusion of his research demonstrated that while scurvy could not be cured with isolated ascorbic acid, consuming it as a whole food had a success record much like the 1996 Chicago Bulls with Michael Jordan.

Instead of making the clear connection between disease and nutrition, medical science continues to round up its unusual suspects and place the blame on innocent accomplices like inherited genetics.

Genetics Are a Predisposition, Not a Predetermination

Since the completion of the Human Genome Project in 2003, we now know that genetics play a very small role in the development and progression of disease. What has a larger impact is the internal environment created by the foods we eat, beverages we drink, stress, and lack of physical activity. These factors create an environment that will either be conducive to health or the feeding ground for disease. A toxic internal environment caused by processed foods, dairy, meat, hormones, refined sugars, dyes, preservatives, artificial colors, heavy metals, stress, and a sedentary lifestyle flips the switch on for genes that code for disease.

The idea that heredity and genes are major determinants of chronic diseases is probably one of the most overstated myths about health. It creates a victim's mind-state as it relates to our well-being instead of the empowered understanding of just how potent our body's healing mechanisms are. When we look at the top killers of Americans, there is no study, physician, or patient who can attest that they have been cured when taking the traditional medicine route. Yes, there are many patients who receive symptom relief, but most often the relief they experience is because the disease has run its course and the body has an innate ability to heal itself. Because modern medicine has been a study of disease instead of healing, naturally more disease has been created. Listening to a drug commercial, even the healthiest person in the world will begin to feel as though they're sick. Today traditional physicians now have a hypochondriac's urge to diagnose and a linebacker's aggression to prescribe. Take a trip to the doctor's office, and you're bound to get diagnosed with anything ranging from restless legs to Alice in Wonderland syndrome (a real diagnosis by the way). Diagnoses are created, and treatments are developed to address all the symptoms; meanwhile, the disease grows progressively worse. Pretty soon, you'll have conditions for your conditions that need to be treated.

The Cascade of Prescription Drugs

It is a well-known practice in the medical field to use drugs to treat the side effects of other previously prescribed drugs. Diabetes is a perfect example of the failures of medicine. This disease doesn't get nearly the amount of attention heart disease or breast cancer does because it's not as sexy as the aforementioned. Most people are completely unaware that they are either pre-diabetic or diabetic, but that's no surprise considering 70% of diabetics also have America's 'silent killer,' hypertension. As sweet as the disease sounds, it doesn't just impact your blood sugars. Diabetes increases the risk of stroke and heart disease up to four-fold, is the leading cause of blindness, accounts for over 60% of all lower limb amputations, 70% of diabetics will suffer mild to severe nerve damage, and it's the leading cause of end-stage kidney disease.

For men, often the canary in the mine (so to speak) is erectile dysfunction. This is the first sign that shows us circulation has been compromised and nerve damage is on its way. At first, it starts off quite simple: metformin (for blood sugar control) and a little HCTZ ('water pill' for blood pressure), and the patient thinks no harm, no foul. But blood pressure can never be regulated by urination for very long because it also leaves the body in a dehydrated state, so two or three additional medications are eventually added because vascular disease will worsen when the cause goes unaddressed. Blood sugar levels will begin to skyrocket due to increased insulin resistance, so additional oral medications are added on.

Type 2 diabetes slowly begins to transition towards type 1 (insulin required). And because all excess sugar in the body is converted into fat, you now have a cholesterol issue (if you didn't have one before), and so a statin drug is added on. At some point, diabetes becomes the sniper in the tower, picking you off piece by piece.

Next, there's gum disease and tooth decay, followed by degeneration of nerves, so gabapentin is added to your medication bank, and then you begin to lose the sensation in your feet altogether. This is followed by gangrene due to a lack of circulation and increased toxicity.

This is why diabetics are at a high risk for amputations. It is not uncommon to see diabetic patients with as many as 20 medications on their profile and leaving the pharmacy with a grocery bag filled with prescriptions.

Does this sound like the traditional model for 'treatment is working'? Of course not, but as you can see, diabetics are the perfect customers for bottom lines. I can remember being a pharmacy manager, reading through our quarterly profit statements, and diabetic patients were always the pharmacy's top revenue patients. Yet there are numerous studies, patient cases, and testimonies that can be easily referenced to show thousands of patients have been *cured* of diabetes by returning to nature's prescription. I can attest personally to this natural prescription because it most certainly saved me from myself. Considering my father had experienced the majority of those progressions, his mother passed as a result of them, along with my mother's

father. With my family history, I could have easily just tossed in the

towel and embraced the belief that genetics superseded my ability to

heal. Even my physicians had told me that my family history made it

a certainty that I should prepare myself for the same diseases. But

what they saw as a genetic precursor, I saw as inherited *habits*

passed down in the form of poor nutrition and lifestyle.

The Truth About Your Genes

For a moment, let's suspend the scientific mumbo-jumbo and

take a trip to common sense land. If the same DNA is passed on to

me from my grandparents and parents containing the same genetic

material as all my brothers, sisters, cousins, aunts, uncles, and

children, why are these genes linked to disease choosing to express

themselves in *some* but not *all* family members? Now we often hear

of dangerous cancer genes that are passed on and put you at high

risk; however, the truth is, genes do *not* self-activate.

A gene cannot turn itself on or off. Genes are turned on or

off by a process known as *gene regulation*. It is an essential part of

normal cell development. Gene regulation can occur at any point but most often occurs at the level of transcription (when information in a gene's DNA is transferred to messenger RNA to make proteins). This process is initiated by either signals from the environment or from *transcription factors*, which are proteins. Regulation of transcription is the most common form of gene control. When these proteins (transcription factors) are not available to respond to the environmental signal, conventional belief is that a random mutation occurs (unpredictable outcome).

This poses a great contradiction to current medical science: hereditary genes are expressing disease selectively, yet the mutation is random. A more likely model was presented by John Cairns *Adaptive mutations*, which states that genes don't change randomly; it is an environmentally directed mutation as a result of the internal environment created by the patient. The idea that genetics has predetermined a patient's health is old medical science that must be retired because we now know that genes only cause 5% or less of all disease. In addition, modern science has proven that 95% of all cancer has no hereditary linkage. Quite the contrary, 95% of cancer is the result of your rewriting normal genes into cancerous genes as a result of the internal environment you create through lifestyle choices.

The expression of disease is not based solely on a genetic predisposition in chronic diseases but the acidic and toxic environment that turns on these genes that express disease.

So the question becomes, what factors can determine a patient's internal environment? That would be what he or she ingests nutritionally, physically, mentally, and spiritually. Anything that we consume that isn't natural and nourishing is a toxin.

If It's Not a Whole Food, It's a Toxin

Anything we eat that cannot be metabolized, absorbed, assimilated, and its remaining by-products eliminated from the system, becomes a toxin.

Modern processed foods are devoid of fiber and saturated with toxic chemicals that accumulate in your colon as rotting fermenting feces. These toxins produce by-products that leach out into the bloodstream and wreak havoc on your blood vessels, tissues, and organs. Ultimately, some of this waste material will be stored in adipose tissue, creating unwanted belly fat.

In very much the same way we can intoxicate ourselves with alcohol, we do the same with modern foods. As we continue to auto-intoxicate ourselves with these food-like products, our bowels will become obstructed, leading to chronic constipation. This vicious cycle is the seat of disease that is digging an early grave for modern people.

You Have to Be a Scientist and Nutritionist Just to Read Food Labels!

We dig our own graves with spoons and forks when we chose to eat out of boxes, cans, jars, and anything that requires a food label.

Being a chemist, pharmacist, and nutritionist gives me a unique perspective on food labels and drug ingredients. On the one hand, I find it fascinating how both organic and inorganic chemistry creates this beautiful symphony we call life and food. But on the other hand, chemicals used in foods today look more reminiscent of the pharmaceutical industry than agriculture. The vast majority of grocery stores are filled with endless aisles of shelf items with expiration dates that will outlive some of their purchasers. We rarely stop to think how these boxed, bagged, canned, and jarred items remain 'fresh' for so long. In order to understand the labels on these 'Franken-foods,' (named after the crudely assembled monster in the horror novel *Frankenstein)*, you would have to be a chemist and nutritionist.

Luckily for you, I just so happen to be both.

The food industry goes to great lengths to ensure that processed foods maintain their color, texture, taste, and especially shelf life. This is how a food product that should contain only two or three ingredients ends up with a laundry list of chemical names you can barely pronounce. Everything from preservatives, dyes, artificial colors, flavor enhancers, and refined sugars are added to hi-jack your taste buds and increase company bottom lines.

The meat industry is worst because packaged meats don't require ingredient labels when they most definitely should. Hormones, antibiotics, and genetically modified organisms are fed to livestock, which subsequently ends up in all animal products, including the dairy products you feed your family. Often these animals are ridden with disease because of the poor living conditions they're subjected to, and these diseases will also end up on your plate.

The Toxins Accumulate

To add fuel to the fire, we layer ourselves with toxic hygienic and cosmetic products that seep into our skins and get into our bloodstream. This is how we intoxicate ourselves literally to death with daily doses of seemingly harmless products that steal away hours, days, and years of our lives in such a gradual fashion they remain undetected.

Our liver and kidneys become saturated with chemicals, and our guts are constipated with backed up sewage. Our health is vitally connected to our ability to eliminate waste from our bodies. Even if we consumed the healthiest foods in the world, chronic constipation would cause those foods to rot and become toxic. Once the body reaches its toxic threshold, disease will most certainly appear. If the toxins accumulate in the knees and joints, then we call it rheumatoid arthritis. Accumulation in the colon, we call it colitis, and in the kidneys, we call it nephritis. All of these signal the initial signs of disease, which is *inflammation*. The inflammation is directly correlated to an inflammatory and toxic diet. This unchecked toxicity will eventually destroy the tissue beyond repair, as is the case with type 1 diabetes and the pancreas.

The great news is that as long as the tissue has not been significantly compromised, the body's healing mechanisms are capable of reversing the disease when the offending toxins are removed from the diet. But even if that weren't the case, it's never too late to enjoy the fruits of the labor from embracing a whole-foods, plant-based lifestyle. Despite the overwhelming evidence to support the benefits of going green, our willingness to hold on to myths about unhealthy foods is why we continue to be the sickest and most obese country in the world.

Other Nations Have Taken Action

In my travels abroad, I noticed another trend. I noticed that not only were many of the food products in America not available outside the U.S., but many of them were banned because many of the ingredients are considered toxic in other nations. There are several hundred chemicals added to American products. Many of these products are banned in most developed nations because they contain chemicals that have been deemed detrimental to their citizens' health.

Here are just a few of the noteworthy unsavory chemicals that we could be handing ourselves doses of on a daily basis:

- Atrazine was banned in Europe in 2003, including Switzerland, where it is manufactured. A UC Berkley professor found that atrazine chemically castrates and feminizes wildlife, and it also lowered the immunity in both wildlife and laboratory rodents. The study also found that the chemical induced breast and prostate cancer, with studies in human populations demonstrating a similar correlation. Used as a weed killer, the chemical has also become a common drinking water contaminant, seeping into our food supply. Despite this overwhelming information, the U.S. Environmental Protection Agency still allows its use.

- The FDA also approved the use of the arsenic-based drugs Roxarsone and Nitarsone, which are used in animal feed (poultry, turkey, and pork) to control infection, increase weight, and make the meat appear more reddish in appearance. The FDA contends these products are safe because they are the organic form of arsenic, which is less toxic than the inorganic form known to be carcinogenic. However, further scientific data has shown that the organic form converts to the inorganic form in tissues, which has been found in elevated levels in store purchased chicken. The manure of those animals also contains inorganic arsenic, which eventually migrates into the soil where it contaminates both water and American rice crops.

By the way, the European Union has never approved this product for safe usage in animal feed.

- The Trojan horse of all chemicals that slips by under our noses undetected are antibiotics. Did you know that 80% of all antibiotics in the U.S. are purchased to feed to livestock animals? These animals are commonly fed antibiotics to prevent disease development and to promote growth. These antibiotics are then passed along to you when you consume meat.

  It is my professional opinion that this also contributes to antibiotic resistance and the development of 'superbugs.' This is a huge medical issue because now there are infectious organisms that no antibiotic is capable of treating.

- Fluoride is shrouded in the cloak of health and prevention even as 185 million citizens are receiving massive amounts in the form of tap water and dental products. Fluoride has been credited with tooth cavity treatment and prevention; however, there are a number of intricacies that should be revealed to discover how public health policy was shaped and formed around this chemical.

The top concern is that the safety standards for water fluoridation in America are based on antiquated science. The first suggestion to fluoridate water can be traced back to a researcher named Gerald Cox of the Mellon Institute of Industrial Research. This suggestion was prompted by Francis Frary, who was a director of an aluminum laboratory. Frary was concerned about the deleterious effects of fluoride on aluminum plant workers, so he asked Cox to look at the proposed benefits of using fluoride for dental cavities.

For some background, the Mellon Institute was a leading proponent of asbestos, which we all now know today is carcinogenic. To protect companies from negligent lawsuits, the Institute repeatedly produced data stating that mesothelioma was not connected to asbestos.

The scientific community is well aware of the catastrophic health effects of fluoride. A quote from the US Department of Agriculture in 1970 states: "Airborne fluorides have caused more worldwide damage to domestic animals than any other air pollutant."

Here's a quote from 1983 by Dr. Leonard Weinstein of Cornell University: "Certainly there has been more litigation on alleged damage to agriculture by fluoride than all other pollutants combined."

At the forefront of the water fluoridation movement was a prominent scientist, Harold Hodge, who adamantly vouched for its safety during the 1950s and 1960s. However, this is the same scientist who was later discovered to be the team leader in the "Human Radiation Experiment," injecting patients with radiation (plutonium) in conjunction with the University of Rochester. A book called *The Plutonium Files* was written detailing the experiment.

Harold Hodge was also the chief toxicologist of the Manhattan Project, which required massive amounts of fluoride for the atomic weapons program and eventually led to many lawsuits as a result of collateral damage during the assembling of the weapons.

Dr. William Marcus, a senior science advisor for the Environmental Protection Agency Office of Water, discovered that the studies conducted on fluoridation of water had been rigged and all the markers for cancer had been downgraded to obscure the correlation of fluoride as a cancer-causing agent in water.

With the number of litigations and toxic effects to workers for companies like Alcoa, US Steel, and others, you might wonder how water fluoridation laws got passed. This 'engineered consent' undoubtedly was the work of the 'Machiavelli of Public Relations' during this period, Edward Bernays, who was hired by the National Institute of Dental Research. In the United States, 67% of the U.S. water supply is fluoridated, while in comparison, 98% of Europe has *banned* water fluoridation.

In addition to water fluoridation, municipal water has been found to contain prescription drugs, heavy metals, and chlorine. The entire modern world is littered with toxins that chip away at our immunity and well-being, and now the food supply is being hijacked!

Fake GMO Food

Food is now being disguised in health with genetically modified organisms (GMO) and passed off as nutrition. The food industry and American government have assured the people that this synthetic food is safe; however, more than thirty European nations have banned this food. And now China and the largest country in the world, Russia, have produced studies that contradict the data provided in the United States. The legislation protecting the masked use of GMO ingredients in American foods is The Safe and Accurate Food Labeling Act of 2015.

The irony of the name has called for opponents of GMOs to rename the bill The Deny Americans the Right to Know (DARK) Act.

This Act was a vendetta against legislation passed in Vermont, Connecticut, and Maine initially requiring GMO labeling on food labels. The Act was created to unravel labeling laws that these states had already implemented as public policy. And despite the fact that here in the U.S. the studies have been mixed as to whether GMOs are safe, the act itself takes away the consumer's right to know whether or not they're eating foods that contain GMOs. This contradicts a 2012 Mellman Group poll that found 91% of American consumers wanted GMOs labeled and a recent CBS/New York Times poll found that 53% of consumers would not purchase foods that were genetically modified.

To understand the true plight of the issue in America, GMOs are present in 80% of conventional processed food and 90% of all soy and corn products.

In a later chapter, GMOs will be further discussed to reveal their impact on health and society as a whole.

Our connection with food on a cultural, social, and emotional level makes it difficult for us to accept a radical change in the things we eat. The foods we eat today look and smell like the foods our grandparents ate, but the majority are imposters at best. The majority of conventional foods are engineered with addiction; so, even when we want to change, it feels impossible to do so.

We can't see the connection between what we eat and the disease in our bodies because most often we *don't want* to see it. Then there are others who are searching for real answers, and they only find lies and myths that lead them right back to where they started.

The China Study

One of the greatest collections of data establishing the link between disease and nutrition is The China Study. It is perhaps the most comprehensive study on nutrition and its connection to disease ever done. The study was conducted over a 20-year period spanning 1978–1997.

Here are just a few parameters that will help you understand why this study was exceptional:

- It included 367 variables, each of which were measured by multiple methods when possible. For example, iron was measured by six different methods, riboflavin (vitamin B2) by three, and so on.

- Sixty-five counties in China were examined, each of which included two separate villages and 100 villagers (over 6,500 adult samples) who completed a battery of questionnaires related to lifestyle and diet, blood tests, urine samples, and more. The populations were stable; an average of 93–94% of the men were born in the village and 89% of women.

- The data was collected over the course of 20 years with the help of surveyors who visited 30% of the test subjects.

- At the completion of the study, there were over 8,000 statistically significant associations between lifestyle, diet, and disease variables.

What made this study unique when compared to all other nutritional studies were the dietary characteristics in rural China. All other studies related to nutrition and its link to disease examined test subjects who were consuming a Western diet rich in processed foods, dairy, unrefined grains, and heavy meat content. This variable remained true even in cases where vegetarians were included in the study because 90% of vegetarians shifted their diet from meat to consuming large quantities of milk, cheese, and eggs. Some still consumed fish and poultry.

The conclusions of the 20-year study were alarming:

- Heart disease can be reversed by embracing a plant-based lifestyle.

- Increased consumption of animal protein and its by-products (dairy: eggs, cheese, milk, butter, etc.) shows a *direct correlation* with increased risk for all chronic diseases.

- Animal protein promotes elevated cholesterol and cancer growth.

In the next chapter, let's explore how animal protein promotes disease.

3.

The Protein Myth

If you think you cannot build muscle on bananas, I challenge you to pick a fight with an ape.
— Garth Davis, M.D., author of Proteinaholic

Many people have a love affair with meat that borders addiction and obsession. The very thought of not having meat during one meal, let alone an entire day, sends them into a frenzy as if you were asking them to stop breathing.

It has to make you wonder why a simple request creates so much anxiety.

At one point in my life, I wouldn't have responded any differently. Yet, despite the fact that I began my plant-based journey in 2011, and here I am, alive, well, and fit, people still don't believe you can survive, much less thrive, on a plant-based lifestyle.

Somehow, protein has become the first and last conversation whenever there is any discussion on the topic of nutrition. Most people embrace the idea that because we are made mostly of muscle, protein is much more significant than any other nutrient.

But when did the words 'meat,' 'muscle,' and 'protein' become synonymous?

And is animal protein really the best source of protein we can have?

Let's address these questions.

In 1838, the Dutch chemist Gerardus Mulder first discovered the chemical structure of proteins. The word 'protein' itself comes from the Greek word *protease,* meaning 'of prime importance.' This was a fitting description, considering it was also discovered that the muscles, skin, and organs are primarily made of proteins.

Proteins are made of varying combinations of twenty *amino acids*, of which eight are called 'essential' because they *must* come from the food you eat (nine for children).

The other twelve can be made by your body.

These twenty amino acids are combined in several thousand chemical permutations that alter the functionality of the protein.

Some of these functions include: enzymes essential for biochemical reactions like digestion, contractile proteins responsible for movement, antibodies that defend the body against foreign invaders, hormones like insulin that regulate glucose (sugar) metabolism, structural proteins like collagen and elastin in tendons and ligaments, and proteins that transport hemoglobin which carries oxygen through the blood.

No one can dispute the supreme importance of protein in all life. However, the belief that because our muscles are made of proteins, we're required to eat massive amounts of animal protein to maintain and build muscle, is a *total myth*.

Prior to the industrialization of our food supply, meat was crowned king because there was a time when only the rich, wealthy, and royalty could afford it. During these times, obesity and opulence were viewed as symbols of wealth and health. Even in America, up until the 1950s, the vast majority of Americans ate meat only on occasions like Sunday dinners and birthdays because it wasn't affordable and wasn't yet so deeply ingrained in our cultural tradition.

Protein is without a doubt the most highly complex of all nutritional sources. There is a much higher energy requirement for digestive elimination of protein than any other macronutrients. Fruits can be easily processed in 20 minutes on an empty stomach, most vegetables, in 60 minutes, and whole grains and legumes can take up to two hours.

Animal protein, however, takes a minimum of five hours to be processed. But this is only if it's a suitable portion size on an empty stomach, not when in combination with other foods. When meat is eaten with other complex macronutrients, the digestive time in the stomach will significantly increase due to the stomach attempting to metabolize proteins, fats, and carbohydrates simultaneously with both acidic and alkaline digestive juices, which will essentially neutralize themselves. This undigested food will then be passed on into the small intestines unfit for assimilation and utilization, and as a result will begin to rot and ferment, releasing methane gas and other toxins into the body, and creating disease instead of providing the intended nourishment for health.

Because of this improper combining of food, most Western societies are constipated, overfed, and malnourished. As a case in point, the first recommendation by the United States Department of Agriculture (USDA) for protein requirements was a whopping 125 grams per day, while today that requirement has been reduced to about 55 grams per day.

Allow me to explain why even this reduced requirement is overstated. The cells in our body are in a constant state of synthesis and breakdown of the body's proteins. The proteins that are broken down are reduced back to their building block component amino acids and returned to circulation. Some of these amino acids are used to synthesize new proteins, some are used for energy, and others are eliminated.

This continuous recycling of proteins in the body is referred to as protein turnover.

Roughly 70%, or 200 grams, of the 300 grams of protein synthesized in the body daily is recycled. This is why our true biological requirement for dietary protein is so little.

In addition, the human body only loses twenty-three grams of protein daily via perspiration, urination, hair loss, defecation, and skin shedding. This is not even equivalent to one ounce, yet it's common dinner etiquette to eat a nine-ounce steak and call it protein replacement.

The claims of danger related to low dietary protein are so farfetched that I can only think of two related medical conditions that exist, marasmus and kwashiorkor, and these conditions are virtually non-existent in Western societies. And no studies have ever confirmed either vegetarians or vegans contracting these conditions.

What is of massive importance is that proteins are *assembled in the body from amino acids*, not from complete proteins. All dietary protein must be digested and then broken down into its amino acid blocks for utilization. Animal protein is dead, denatured by cooking, and in the form of a complete protein, not an amino acid. When we eat animal protein, our body has to break those complete proteins down into amino acids, sift through the remaining by-products to determine what is usable, and then safely eliminate the remaining waste.

This is the bottom line:

- Your body does *not* use protein directly from food.
- Our bodies make proteins from commonly available amino acids.

- *It does not care where these amino acids come from.* The amino acids from a lion's heart (to use a romantic 'warrior' example) are exactly the same amino acids you get from ordinary chickpeas. To your body, they're all equally good raw materials.

The thing to remember is that in many other ways, foods like chickpeas don't create the toxic by-products that animal protein does.

The artificial synthesizing of products like creatinine and its protein peers for bodybuilding and high protein fad diets are not only misaligned with nature but detrimental to health. Let me assure you; there are no shortcuts to massive muscle gains and weight loss that are not without risks.

However, you can rest assured there are natural options to both that are long-term in nature and can provide the same results minus the risk.

Jim Morrison, who is a former Mr. America, Mr. USA, Olympia, and Mr. Universe, is 71 years old and still looks primed for competition. He's vegan and an advocate of a plant-based lifestyle.

Alex Dargatz is famous for winning the World Bodybuilding competition in 2005 after being vegan for five years.

Billy Simmonds won Mr. Natural Universe in 2009 and also is vegan.

Olympic medal-winning track star Carl Lewis claimed that his best years of competing were when he first embraced a plant-based vegan lifestyle.

Also on the list of non-meat eating notables from history are Leonardo da Vinci, Benjamin Franklin, Mark Twain, Albert Einstein, and Steve Jobs. Not a bad list to be on. Most of the current and past science on protein is not based on what nature demonstrates. Around the world, when we study blue-zone populations who live the longest with the highest quality of health, we find a plant-based lifestyle at the center of their fountain of youth. What we also discover is that heart disease, the number one killer of humans, is virtually non-existent for these populations.

Animal Meat and Organ Damage

So how is our consumption of meat directly connected to heart disease and other problems?

Animal protein is the sole source of saturated fat, the same type of fat that clogs arteries and leads to cardiovascular disease. Consumption of animal protein has been shown not only to cause heart disease but can also alter the function and structure of the kidneys.

Chronic kidney disease now affects one out of every eight Americans, and 25% of those affected are not even aware. The excessive amount of protein we're consuming puts a tremendous amount of wear and tear on the kidneys, gradually causing the function to decline, and in many cases leading to kidney disease that eventually leads to the need for dialysis.

Excess animal protein increases dietary acid loads, which cause the blood to become acidic. This will ultimately increase renal acid excretion and ammonia production, triggering a condition known as metabolic acidosis.

This is exactly why in practice it's recommended to restrict protein intake to prevent the progression of kidney disease and stones. Restricting protein consumption is the equivalent of removing your foot from the accelerator of a car that's been pressed to the max over an extended period.

When we compare the impact of animal protein versus plant-based proteins, we don't see these effects. As reported in the *Journal of Clinical Investigation,* a comparable amount of plant-based protein demonstrates almost no effect on the kidneys.

The same goes for gout patients. Many types of meats are high purine compounds that elevate uric acid levels in the blood, leading to a gout attack.

These patients often try to negotiate which meats to avoid, but everything from red meat to fish can lead to a flare-up. A good rule of thumb for overall health is animal protein of any kind will have some level of impact on our health. To be clear, animal protein does also include fish and dairy products. The impact of a dramatic reduction in animal protein in one's diet can sometimes bring instant results. When patients with compromised kidney function are switched to a plant-based vegan diet, we witness functional improvement to the kidneys.

Studies have shown that animal protein can trigger an inflammatory response in the kidneys. A 2013 meta-analysis of meat consumption and diabetes published in *Current Diabetes* found that saturated and animal fat intake is associated with elevated insulin levels and insulin resistance. Also, dietary cholesterol, which is primarily found in animal protein, was indicated as a potential risk for type 2 diabetes. Both animal protein and dairy are known to stimulate insulin and burn out the insulin-producing beta cells in the pancreas, which causes type 2 diabetes.

The Epic-Inter Act study "The association of dietary meat consumption and incident of type 2 diabetes" followed 16,835 individuals that were observed for 11.7 years and found that for every 50 grams of animal protein (which would be equivalent to a 1/4 of a chicken breast), there was an 8% increase in risk for type 2 diabetes.

Americans Eat Too Much Meat

The Western diet and those who profit from it have created an insatiable craving for meat built on the foundation of misinformation and propaganda. The average American consumes 200 pounds of meat and 30 pounds of cheese annually. Americans eat more meat per person than any other people on Earth, and we're paying the price in health care bills. As a result, Americans are twice as obese and have twice as much diabetes and nearly triple the cancer rate compared to other countries. Americans are gorging themselves on meat without having ever considered that 800 million people are starving globally while we currently produce enough food to feed 10 billion people, or that 6 million innocent animals are killed every hour for food, or that 15 times more protein could be produced with plants on any given area of land compared to animal protein.

We Were Born to Be Plant Eaters

The same science we use to determine what dinosaurs ate millions of years before human existence we chose to blatantly ignore when it comes to determining what foods were designed for our own biology. Paleobiologists primarily use the teeth and jaws from fossils to determine their diet. Sharp serrated teeth and strong jaw structures are indicative of carnivores to tear into flesh and bite chunks out of meat. The jaw of a carnivore is typically strong enough to break bones. The strength of the jaws can be determined by observing how muscles were attached to bones.

Herbivores had flat, dull, rounded teeth like ours that are exceptional for chewing and grinding plant foods. The fact that our jaws move side to side to assist with grinding when carnivores like an alligator only move up and down in a snapping motion is further proof of this.

Furthermore, a plant eater's saliva is alkaline. Ours specifically is amylase, and its primary function is to break down carbohydrates and starches into their sugar by-products. This biological design is specifically designed to eat and metabolize plant-based foods. Below is a list of plant-based protein sources. I included soy milk, tofu, and soya beans in an attempt not to be biased; however, I do not recommend using these products because all soy products contain natural anti-nutrients and phytoestrogens that can be detrimental to your health long-term. Hemp is the most bioavailable protein source in the world, whether it's compared to plant or animal-based sources. This is because hemp is biologically, in alignment with our digestive system.

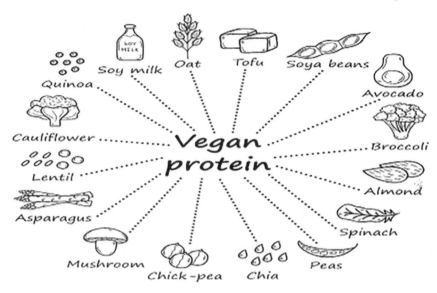

When we look at the physiological make-up of carnivores, we see man contrasts. A carnivore's saliva is acidic in nature, which is required to break down animal protein. The stomach of a carnivore is capable of digesting rotting flesh riddled with bacteria without producing the faintest sign of discomfort. This is primarily because their stomachs produce ten times the amount of hydrochloric acid compared to ourselves and herbivores. This creates a highly acidic environment in the stomach, perfect for digesting proteins at a pH roughly 1−2 (highly acidic). This highly acidic pH makes it nearly impossible for salmonella, E. coli, parasites, worms, or other pathogens to survive during digestion.

For humans and other herbivores, the pH ranges from 4–5. This is why humans must cook their meats. The cooking process denatures the large majority of the proteins, allowing for the moderately acidic stomach to digest foods and kill some of the bacteria and pathogens that may be present.

Let's look further at how anatomy tells us what foods we are made to eat. The small intestine of a carnivore or omnivore (an animal that eats both plants and flesh) is on average 3–6 times the length of their body torso. This anatomical design allows for rapid elimination of acidic foods, like meat, to prevent the digested food from rotting.

In contrast, the small intestines of herbivores are on average 10–11 times the length of the torso. So roughly that's a small intestine comparison of 7–10 feet for carnivores vs. 20–25 feet for herbivores and humans.

The elimination canal or colon of carnivores is short, and its walls are smooth. The colon for herbivores and humans is long, with saclike pouches which make it conducive for prolonged nutrient absorption. This physiological design is a perfect pipeline for the creation of a cesspool-like internal environment when eating meat. It increases the bowel transport time, allowing food to rot and ferment.

When Food Becomes Toxic

When food isn't properly digested, it becomes toxic and begins seeping into the bloodstream, poisoning the body along with the bacteria and other pathogens it creates. Once in the bloodstream, these toxins travel to tissues, vital organs, and joints to manifest themselves as disease. Initially, the body will attempt to eliminate them by the normal elimination routes and also by forming a mucus: via the scalp, it manifests as dandruff; in the head and throat, it becomes a cold; in the lungs, it becomes an upper or lower respiratory tract infection; in the eyes, it becomes glaucoma; in the pancreas, it becomes diabetes; and so on.

This mucus is acidic in nature, so any bacteria, virus, or fungi will flourish there. Acidity and toxins tend to concentrate in the weakest areas of the body. The longer the tissue is exposed to this acidic environment, more of the tissue will become degenerated.

Let's use our common sense for a moment to evaluate if eating animals for muscle really makes sense. In general, people eat cows, pigs, chickens, and fish to get the protein they need for muscle. Don't you find it odd that all of these animals eat a plant-based diet, and yet magically they all have muscle? If you think that's circumstantial, think about this: What do gorillas, elephants, and rhinos eat? They all eat a plant-based diet and are some of the largest and strongest animals on the planet.

Our human DNA is 99% compatible with the chimpanzees. This is why they are often tragically used in clinical trials and studies to observe possible responses to drugs, chemicals, and other stimuli to predict correlated biological response in humans. Their primate cousins, mountain gorillas, can grow to six feet tall and weigh up to 500 pounds. Many experts have estimated that their strength can be up to ten times that of a human. And what does their diet consist of (according to Sea World)? 86% leaves, shoots, and stems; 7% roots; 3% flowers; 2% snails, ants, and grubs.

Nature proves without bias that the idea of animal protein consumption being equivalent to muscle growth is ridiculous.

Making the Change to a Plant-based Lifestyle

I know that if you consume meat, all of this information must be shocking and poking at every shred of your moral fiber, but I can assure you I've experienced all the thoughts you're thinking. *Is it really true?* Do your own research—I encourage you.

But you ask:

I love meat so much; how can I live without the desirable taste of chicken, steak, or fish?

You can, and you will, even more vibrantly once you readjust your taste buds back to their natural settings.

What will I substitute in the place of meat?

There are more plant-based sources of protein than animal-based proteins, and with a ton of delicious recipes to match.

Will the cravings ever go away?

Yes! Actually, you will eventually become repulsed by the thought of eating meat.

How can I explain this decision to my family, friends, and others?

You don't have to explain it. Share the health benefits you received, the impact you're making on our planet, and the compassion you're giving to the other earthlings living on this planet. Then encourage them without judgment to try it for themselves.

Why should I change? I enjoy eating meat, and I'm currently healthy.

Because the meat you're eating, and the amount you're eating is not the same as your grandparents, and your health today doesn't guarantee tomorrow without prevention.

You can do it! I believe in you because I was able to do it. I'm the same guy who decided his reward for graduating pharmacy school would be to go to the Steak House and have a filet mignon anytime I wanted for the sacrifices I made, and the same guy who ate meat during every meal of his life up until the point I decided not to.

If you don't see my personal evolution as inspiring enough, then look at Howard Lyman, a former Montana cattle rancher for four decades who sold his farm and became vegetarian in light of health concerns. He later appeared on the Oprah Winfrey Show and openly talked about the dangers of eating beef, for which he and Oprah were sued by the National Cattlemen's Beef Association.

Today Mr. Lyman is not only vegan but an avid animal rights advocate and author on related subjects. He has said, "My life experience has given me a better understanding of what is happening, and what a mistake it is to believe, there is anything called 'humane' slaughter. Animals have families and feelings, and to think that kindness before killing them is an answer is totally wrong. Humans have no need for animal products. And when we consume animal products, we're not just killing the animals. In the long run, we're killing the planet, and ourselves. No animal has to die in order for me to live. And that makes me feel good."

The Impact of the Livestock Industry on the World

The single greatest infliction on health and the global environment is the consumption of animal protein and animal agriculture. The live stocking of animals and animal agriculture have become the leading causes of deforestation, pollution, rainforest destruction, greenhouse gases, species extinction, and water consumption. The reassuring lie that fossil fuels and carbon dioxide are our greatest threats, has been replaced by an inconvenient truth among staunch meat eaters and the $100 billion

service providers.

The documentary *Cowspiracy* exposes the global destruction

caused by factory farming and reveals the enormous lump hidden

beneath the rug by the world's leading environmental agencies and

the animal agriculture industry. According to the Worldwatch

Institute, livestock and their byproducts account for at least 51% of

all worldwide greenhouse gas emissions. One of the primary

attributors to this fact is because methane (yes, from cow farts) has a

global warming potential 86 times that of carbon dioxide and is up

to 100 times more destructive in a twenty-year time frame. And these

emissions are projected to increase by 80% by the year 2050 to keep

up with our demand for animal protein and our growing population.

To put this reality into perspective, even if we completely cut

the use of fossil fuels and converted to renewal sustainable options,

we still will exceed our carbon dioxide limit by the year 2030.

This is all attributed to the live stocking of animals. These

animals and the grains grown to feed them occupy 45% of the

earth's total land, and in the U.S., half of the land is used for animal

agriculture.

Suggestions like carpooling, eating less meat, and turning off lights are meaningless acts to solve a gigantic global issue. The collateral damage of this industry isn't limited to our atmosphere, but overgrazing has also desertified 1/3 of the planet and destroyed 91% of the Amazon. Folks, Amazon basin, is the equivalent of the Earth's lungs, producing the air you and I breathe. Every second, up to two acres of rainforest are destroyed, and 137 plant, animal, and insect species are lost daily.

And if you think this has gone unnoticed, just refer to the 1,100 land activists who have been killed in Brazil in protest of this injustice in the past 20 years. One was Sister Dorothy Stang, a missionary nun who was gunned down in Brazil for speaking out against the cattle ranching industry in 2005.

These atrocities are not only being committed on land, but the insult has been taken to the seas. Each year, some 100 million tons of fish are pulled from the ocean. National Geographic researchers say it's possible by the year 2048 we could have a fishless ocean.

4.

Ditch the Dairy

The human body has no more need for cows' milk than it does for dogs' milk, horses' milk, or giraffes' milk.
—Michael Klaper, MD

The very thought of the word 'dairy' probably creates picturesque mental images of cows peacefully grazing green pastures and musclebound athletes flexing their biceps as a representation of strong bones. This is no doubt due to the barrage of commercials we grew up watching—like 'Got Milk?'—and decades of advocacy for dairy in the U.S. Department of Agriculture's (USDA) food pyramids. Nutritionists and healthcare professionals corroborated these suggestions by counseling every patient on the importance of dairy providing both calcium and vitamin D to grow strong bones.

The litany of commercial advertisements advocating for the consumption of milk for the benefit of strong bones is ingrained in the fabric of western societies.

But the questions raised by the Harvard School of Public Health is whether we need as much calcium as recommended and if dairy products are the best sources.

The USDA spent $550 million to convince the American public that "Beef—It's what's for dinner" and "Milk does a body good." It has to make you wonder, *What logic did we use to replace human breast milk all together with cow's milk?*

In nature, every other mammal begins lactation (milk production) in the mammary glands immediately after giving birth. With the exception of humans, all other mammals are weaned off milk after infancy. But ironically, we've developed a lifelong dependency on cow's milk. You'll never see an ape drinking elephant's milk or a puppy drinking cat's milk. Yet, for some strange and slightly deranged reason, we find it kosher to drink cow's milk.

It seems almost moronic to believe that breast milk could be swapped out as an even exchange for cow's milk as if the two were the same. Cow's milk is specifically designed to super-size an 85-pound baby calf into a 500-pound cow in less than a year. We're genetically and structurally incompatible with cows, yet we've made cow's milk the elixir of life for strong bones.

Nature engineered every mammal's milk suitable for its own specific developmental needs. The enzymes, hormones, sugars, and protein composition in cow's milk are not even close to human breast milk.

This is largely why dairy is one of the most common food allergies. This creates an immune reaction that leads to inflammation and mucus production. This immune response often leads to ear infections, respiratory issues, post-nasal drip, sinusitis, nasal congestion, rashes, hives, eczema, and digestive problems. Take a look at these symptoms and think about how common they are in children. Ditching dairy is my number one recommendation for parents with children suffering from asthma and chronic ear infections.

Casein and Whey: The Gruesome Twosome

The proteins casein and whey found in dairy are primarily responsible for our body's allergic reactions.

Casein is the solid portion of milk that creates curdles, while whey makes up the remaining liquid portion. The primary difference in how these two proteins impact our health is how they are digested.

Whey protein is rapidly digested and absorbed into the blood, causing a spike in insulin production and eventually insulin growth factor (IGF-1). During childhood, IGF-1 is a critical growth hormone for normal development, but for adults, it can cause the production, proliferation, and metastasis of cancerous cells. Essentially, IGF-1 is rocket fuel for cancer growth. It doesn't matter if you buy milk organic or raw, it will still contain these cancer-promoting hormones.

The more predominant form of protein in milk is casein. Casein is an insoluble protein that forms clumps that are slowly peeled away in the stomach, causing its digestion to take up to several hours. Dr. T. Colin Campbell, author and researcher of The China Study, said his research concluded, "Casein, which makes up

87% of milk protein, is the most relevant cancer promoter ever identified."

Both breast and cow's milk contain casein; however, it's 300 times more abundant in cow's milk. The slow digestion of these proteins in our stomachs produces morphine-like compounds called *casomorphins*. The compounds are capable of stimulating the release of histamines, which is why 75% of the world's population has some form of reaction to dairy. Casomorphins enter the bloodstream, then travel to the brain and attach to opiate receptors, producing similar effects of opioid drugs, like morphine. The same compounds are present in human breast milk at significantly lower concentrations and appear to have an evolutionary purpose. According to Dr. Neal Barnard, author of *The Cheese Trap* and founder of the Physicians Committee for Responsible Medicine, "It appears that the opiates from mother's milk produce a calming effect on the infant and, in fact, may be responsible for a good measure of the mother-infant bond. It turns out that it's not all lullabies and cooing. Psychological bonds always have a physical underpinning. Like it or not, mother's milk has a drug-like effect on the baby's brain that ensures that the baby will bond with Mom and continue to nurse and get the nutrients all babies need. But like heroin and codeine, casomorphins in cheese retard intestinal movement and have an antidiarrheal effect. The opiate effect may be why adults often find that cheese can be constipating and addictive, just as opiate painkillers are."

Why You Should Avoid Cheese

It appears that addiction is engineered even into breast milk. However, the concentration of these morphine-like compounds in cheese is like milk on steroids.

To make one block of cheese requires ten gallons of milk. The majority of water and whey protein is removed from milk during the process. What's left behind is a concentrated block of fat and casein protein filled with opiate compounds. This is why for most people who've transitioned to a plant-based lifestyle, kicking the cheese habit was much harder even compared to meat.

I won't go as far to compare our addiction to cheese to the prescription opioid crisis here in America, but I don't think it's a stretch to say cheese has a devastating impact on our overall health as a country. After all, cheese seems to be the perfect recipe for heart disease. It's the number one source of saturated fat in the American diet, has the cholesterol equivalent of a steak, and is one of the leading sources of sodium of all foods.

What makes ditching dairy so complicated now is that it's not just in dairy products anymore. It's hidden in baked goods, candy, pizza crust, and even medications. A quick glance at the label of products marketed as vegan or non-dairy, and you will often find hidden dairy in the form of casein and soy lecithin. Casein can also be found in adhesives, glues, and plastics. This is why the popular brand Elmer's Glue, commonly used by school children, has a cow on the front label. Do you really want to drink or eat something that promotes cancer and is capable of making glue in your digestive tract?

Inside the human stomach, milk proteins coagulate and create difficult-to-digest curdles that make a fine paste throughout the digestive tract. This retards the absorption of nutrients and hampers the immune system.

The nutritional value in cow's milk is lost through the process of pasteurization, which heats the milk at a temperature of 161 degrees Fahrenheit. This kills all nutrients and denatures many of the proteins. This process also degrades the calcium, which becomes far less absorbable due to it being engulfed by a casein matrix. This is why milk is then 'fortified' with calcium from synthetic sources. While synthetic sources of calcium will falsely normalize your lab values, therapeutically you will still be deficient.

How to Get Calcium

Dark green leafy vegetables such as kale, Swiss chard, spinach, collard greens, and mustard greens are great sources of calcium. The daily recommended requirement for calcium is based on the average absorption of 25%. This does not take into consideration the diet of the vegan and raw enthusiast, who will absorb at much high rates due to a cleaner and healthier digestive tract.

Sesame seeds are also packed with calcium. Just one tablespoon provides 88 mg (one cup is 1,404 mg). But since the likelihood of anyone having a cup of sesame seeds is zero to none, tahini, a Mediterranean sesame seed paste, is an ideal source that can be used in a variety of recipes like delicious salad dressings.

Another alternative is adding one cup of flaxseed to a green smoothie, salad, or collard greens, which provides 266 mg of calcium per cup.

If your sweet tooth calls for a more intriguing option, fruits are bursting with calcium.

So if you're eating dark green leafy vegetables, fruits, and seeds daily, you will never have to concern yourself with a calcium deficiency.

Vitamin D

Ironically, vitamin D isn't a vitamin at all but a hormone. But because of its significance and the body's inability to self-synthesize this hormone, it is referred to as a fat-soluble vitamin required from food or supplements.

Or is it?

Vitamin D is also made by the skin's exposure to UV rays from the sun. The plants we eat receive the same vitamin D via the same photons. For a fair skinned person, exposing the face, hands, and back without sunscreen for 20 minutes four times a week would be an adequate dose for health. That's free vitamin D, with a priceless amount of health in exchange.

Vitamin D deficiency is linked to several chronic diseases like cancer and cardiovascular disease. This is because vitamin D is essential to every cell in the body.

Like calcium, it is synthetically supplemented into dairy products. One cup of milk only has 100 international units of vitamin D. You would have to drink 100 cups of milk daily to prevent a deficiency. Dairy products are also highly acidic. When we consume acidic foods like dairy, they cause our blood to become acidic. In order to restore alkalinity in the blood, the body will begin pulling from its alkaline reserves. The irony is, the body pulls calcium from the bones to restore the blood pH. So, inevitably, this mineral leaching will lead to osteoporosis because 99% of all calcium is stored in the bones and teeth.

I know what you're probably thinking: There's so much conflicting data as to whether dairy is a source of health or a producer of disease; most people are caught in between the two like a deer in headlights. This is why I always encourage you to do your own research and ask better questions. Always find out who funded a particular study. Determine if they stand to benefit from the study. An agency receiving funding from the dairy industry, an institution of higher learning receiving a grant from a pharmaceutical company, a professor at a university seeking tenure, or a policymaker who's been heckled and bribed by a lobbyist? The China Study, for instance, was a partnership between Cornell University, Oxford University, and the Chinese Academy of Preventative Medicine. The project was jointly funded by both universities and the Chinese government. The Emperor of China was dying of cancer at the time of the study and was seeking real answers. Does this sound like a study you could probably trust?

There's a dysfunctional system making a living off the public's misery, and to a certain degree, we're being asked to be co-conspirators in our own demise. Did you know that we as taxpayers subsidize dairy products to the tune of $38 billion annually? This subsidizes both the dairy and meat industry, as opposed to $17 million spent to subsidize fruits and vegetables. So the federal government's food guidelines are urging us to eat more fruits and vegetables and reduce foods that are cholesterol-rich (which are meat and dairy products), yet the tax funding is completely contradictory. These subsidies include emergency supplemental 'market loss' payments of $1 billion to compensate dairy producers for low prices between 1999 and 2001.

As a caveat, in 2002, Congress enacted the Milk Income Loss Contract (MILC) program to make these compensations permanent, which provides direct payments to dairy farmers when the average monthly price of milk falls below standard pricing. In the past fifteen years, only one-third of American farmers actually received these subsidies, which were valued at $100 billion, while the remaining two-thirds went to large corporations.

The USDA and the Beef Lobby

Our system encourages the growth of factory farms and strangles the local farmer and surrounding community. With a name like United States Department of Agriculture (USDA), you would think this agency would be primarily pushing fruits and vegetables; however, the bulk of their advertisement has always been for beef and dairy. They are primarily financed by the meat industry and educated by nutritional scientists who are bankrolled by the same industry. The recommendations are not evidence-based, which can be easily seen today on our kids' lunch menus. They now consider pizza and packets of ketchup a vegetable. Do frozen processed pizza and ketchup laden with high fructose corn syrup remotely resemble any vegetable?

The Harvard University School of Public Health concluded, "The USDA's recommendations are based on out-of-date science and influenced by people with business interests." The USDA began endorsing the campaign of a non-profit that promoted 'Meatless Monday,' and the slogan suggested going meatless on Mondays. The support for the campaign was posted on their July 2014 edition of the USDA's internal 'Green Headquarters' newsletter, advocating for employees to refrain from eating meat in the cafeteria on Mondays.

The newsletter has since been removed.

You might ask, "What would prompt the USDA to recall its support?" Following the USDA's support, its largest financier, National Cattlemen's Beef Association (NCBA), posted this statement to its website: "This move by the USDA should be condemned by anyone who believes agriculture is fundamental to sustaining life on this planet." The president of NCBA, J.D.

Alexander, went further to say, "When it comes to health, beef has an amazing story to tell. Beef is a naturally nutrient-rich food helping you get more nutrition from the calories you take in."

One thing that's for sure is, if beef (cow) were able to tell its story, it would be more of a horror film than a happy ending.

Our citizens are drowning themselves in beef, chicken, pork, and fish raised in factory farms that drench these poor animals with antibiotics, growth hormones, and chemicals. Not to mention the diseases manifested as a result of the poor farming conditions. This consistent miseducation of the public with crooked science and manipulative financial tactics, is the foundation of why America is the most obese and sickest country in the world.

Despite having the best medical technology, America is ranked 37th in the world's health polls. These numbers don't lie. But some do like the dairy industry's ingenious use of numbers that often tricks you into buying a seemingly healthier product. In calculating nutritional values for dairy products, weight is used instead of the total number of calories. With milk, for instance, if we used calories instead of weight, a more accurate analysis of nutritional value is discovered. We find that whole milk is 49% fat (that's half of what you drink), and that 2% milk (the proposed 'healthier' alternative) is 35% fat. What the heck? Nutritionally, 2% milk is just as bad as whole milk.

Your liver naturally makes cholesterol as you sleep, which is essentially the creation of hormones and a number of other important functions. This cholesterol is sufficient for the body's needs, so all other dietary cholesterol consumed in meat, dairy, and processed foods products in the form of saturated fats ends up creating occluded plaque in your coronary arteries, which leads to heart disease—the *number one* cause of death. The number one killer of humans globally is poor nutritional habits that can be prevented by embracing a plant-based lifestyle.

So ditch the dairy!

5.

The Bitter Truth About Sugar

Sugar feeds cancer cells and stimulates tumor growth. Cancer cells have ten times more insulin receptors than normal cells. —Dr. David Jockers

We have a bittersweet relationship with sugar. Most of us wouldn't disagree that sugar is bad for our health, yet Americans consume an average of 160 pounds of added sugar every year. Let me help put that in perspective: two hundred years ago, the annual consumption per person was 18 pounds. Next time you're in the grocery store, grab 18 pounds of sugar and hold it in your hand if you can just to get a better perspective. Then imagine yourself carrying around 160 pounds up and down the aisles.

It would be a huge understatement to say Americans are in love with sugar, and probably more appropriate to say there's an obsession or borderline addiction. To some extent, we're

programmed to want sugar; after all, glucose is the primary form of

fuel our bodies need for energy to perform the majority of our

biological functions. However, the added sugar we're eating by the

pounds is more of a poison than a love potion.

Throughout this chapter, I'll explain how sugar is directly

related to obesity, heart disease, cancer, lowered immunity,

metabolic syndrome, tooth decay, and how food companies have

cleverly hidden sugar in many of the foods we eat to feed our

addiction. I also explain the dark history of our deep-seated

fascination with our sweet tooth.

First, let me give you some foundation of my philosophy. I

take a holistic approach to every aspect of life, not just healing.

Instead of examining just the part of a whole to treat, like traditional

medicine does, I look at the whole to see how all the parts work in

unison so that I can see how nature heals itself. So when I hear the

word 'sugar,' I understand it in context, not as just a part.

In nature, sugar does not exist alone. It is always taken from

a whole. In very much the same way if I were to remove your heart from your body, you would cease to exist, and your heart would lose purpose and function.

When we refer to sugar as a form of nutrition, it is called glucose. In nature, you will only find glucose as part of a carbohydrate matrix. Glucose is produced as the by-product of carbohydrates being broken down during digestion and is transported in the blood to the brain, muscles, and other critical cells to be utilized as energy. These molecules are called carbohydrates because they contain carbon, hydrogen, and oxygen in the same ratio as water (H_2O), which comprises roughly 75% of the earth and our bodies.

Our Sugar Addiction

Despite this evolutionary propensity towards a sweet tooth, humans did not develop an obsession for the taste of white sugar until the American continents established the sugar industry via slave trade in the Caribbean. In 1537, the first sugar refinery was established in Germany, primarily for sugar cane. Up until the middle of the 18th century, sugar was considered a luxury and commonly referred to as 'The White Gold.' By the 1700s, the

average person consumed four pounds of sugars annually; by the
1800s, about 18 pounds; and then in the 1900s, it spiked to 90
pounds. By the year 2009, Americans were gorging themselves on
170 pounds of sugar annually. That's nearly 1/2 pound of sugar
daily!

This increase has been marked by similar trends in health
decline and disease. In 1660, Britain discovered that sugar was so
profitable it passed the Navigation Act of 1660 preventing transport
of sugar outside of British territories, and by 1662, they were
importing 16 million pounds of sugar. Just three years later, London
was swept by the bubonic plague, and over 68,000 people died.

In 1674, the first case of diabetes mellitus was mentioned in
the British *Pharmaceutice Rationalis*.

By 1792 the Anti-Saccharite Society had been formed in
Europe to educate society on the dangers of sugar to the public's
health. In 1812, Napoleon Bonaparte awarded Benjamin Delessert
with the Legion of Honor for discovering how to process beets, a
root vegetable, into sugar to replace the dependency on sugar cane,
which was the primary source of sugar coming from British colonies
in the Caribbean. Sugar cane cannot be grown in harsh weather

conditions that are prevalent in Europe because it requires a tropical environment as compared to the beets.

By 1900, America took the lead in worldwide sugar consumption, overtaking Britain. At the turn of the century, the top two killers of Americans were influenza and pneumonia at number one, and tuberculosis at number two. In 1918, between 50 and 100 million people died worldwide during the influenza pandemic, making it one of the deadliest natural disasters in history.

High Fructose Corn Syrup

Here's another sweet moment in history. In 1970, due to the political climate and trade restrictions in cane sugar producing countries, high fructose corn syrup (HFCS) was introduced to the US food system. It had been invented in Japan by a scientist, Yoshiyuki Takasaki, in 1966. In an attempt to win political points with voters, Richard Nixon instructed his secretary of agriculture to come up with ways to make food cheaper. HFCS made its way into the American food supply because it was cheaper and sweeter than table sugar.

Then in the 1980s, in response to the fat-free fad pushed by the American Heart Association and USDA, it was added to virtually every processed food to compensate for the removal of fat. But everyone failed to do the necessary research to determine what was this Franken-sugar we had decided to add to everything.

What is important for you to know is the fructose in HFCS is nothing like glucose, the sugar your body uses for energy. It can't even be compared to the fructose in fruits. No form of added sugar can be compared to sugars in whole foods. Whether added sugar is extracted from cane or beets or created in a lab like HFCS, it always requires chemical processing. What may be more confusing is when we look at the sugar composition of most fruits, which is typically 42% to 50% fructose, and the remaining is glucose, while table sugar, by comparison, is 50/50, so it appears no harm no foul because the ratios are so similar.

But I can assure you all sugar isn't created equal, especially HFCS.

Dangers of Fructose in HFCS
Fructose is 7 times more likely to create AGEs (Advanced Glycation End-Products)
Causes Weight Gain and Obesity
Elevates risk for Type-2 Diabetes
Can lead to High Blood Pressure
Elevates Bad Cholesterol
Unlike Natural Sugar, HFCS does not suppress hunger
Unlike Natural Sugar, HFCS does not stimulate insulin release
Has the same impact on the liver as alcohol abuse
HFCS leads to Mercury Exposure

HFCS is extracted from 'dent' corn, which is not edible unless it goes through a refining process. This industrial food product is far from natural. The process by which HFCS is extracted from corn stalks is so secret that Cargill and Archer Daniels Midland refuses to allow investigative reporters to review the process.

The word 'high' refers specifically to the high concentration of fructose compared to glucose in an unbound form.

Metabolizing Sugars

It is of importance to note that the human body metabolizes fructose and glucose very differently. While virtually every cell in the body can metabolize glucose, the liver cells are alone in their capacity to metabolize fructose. This fact alone should raise a red flag, as the liver is the primary organ for metabolizing all toxins and poisons that enter the body. When we consume HFCS in any food, this sugar goes undigested and rapidly enters the bloodstream. Unbound fructose in the blood causes a huge spike in blood sugar and insulin, which with prolonged exposure can lead to insulin resistance and diabetes. It then travels to the liver where it stimulates the production of triglycerides and cholesterol. This leads to a condition known as *nonalcoholic fatty liver*. This was virtually nonexistent prior to 1980 (ten years after the introduction of HFCS to the world) but now affects 30% of all adults in developed countries.

In addition to the increased fat deposits, excess fructose causes elevated blood pressure, increased free radical production, promotes fat build up around visceral organs (belly fat), and makes the tissues insulin resistant to the uptake of glucose, causing high blood sugars. According to a 2010 article published in the *New England Journal of Medicine,* elevated insulin levels are a precursor to cardiovascular disease.

Here's another amazing comparison. The US Department of Agriculture (USDA) states that between 1970 and 1990, the consumption of HFCS increased 1,000 percent. This exponential increase is also mirrored by a doubling in the incidence of diabetes to the tune of 350 million since 1980, fueled by an epidemic rise in obesity in the United States.

In the last thirty years, we've also seen a threefold increase in childhood diabetes. This is catastrophic if you realize that before 1980, it was rare to find individuals under the age of thirty with either type 1 or 2 diabetes, and now it's becoming normal to diagnose ten-year-olds with both type 1 and 2 diabetes.

The entire dynamic of our food culture has been stripped of once-standard, naturally-grown foods into fast, cheap, processed pseudo-foods. So, today, instead of children being barraged with advertisements and commercials on a Saturday morning full of cartoons, a countless number of sugary food products race across the screen, manipulating your child's desires. Each is stuffed full of sugary Pied Piper artificial sugars to evoke desperate begging for their purchase. The food industry spends billions of dollars to tantalize children's taste buds with this unnatural sugar as the secret sauce to the crazed loyalty to their products.

HFCS isn't limited to just food products. It just so happens to be 40% of sugar that is added to soft drinks and the drinks that are often called 'juice' but typically contain 3% or less of actual fruit juice.

It is also inserted into white and wheat breads, cereals, snacks that are labeled as healthy, as well as crackers, ketchup, chips, candy bars, salad dressing, and pretty much anything that isn't in the produce section of the supermarket. The Institute for Agriculture and Trade Policy, a non-profit watchdog group, analyzed 55 of the top brand-name foods and found that one-third contained HFCS with trace amounts of mercury. Most recently, the corporations have underhandedly rebranded HFCS as just simply 'fructose' as if it were naturally occurring. This is exactly why public policies like the Dark Act are abominable to the health of the public. Despite the overwhelming amount of evidence and correlation between the introduction of HFCS and the increased prevalence of obesity, diabetes, cancer, and other illnesses, sugars in all forms are still dramatically increasing in our food supplies.

The truth is that without the presence of natural fiber, *all* forms of sugars are acidic. Excess sugar feeds disease in the body. Whether it be diabetes or cancer. This includes some vegetables, especially if the body is already in an acidic state. More specifically, I'm referring to starchy vegetables like peas, carrots, corn, potatoes, and winter squash.

When unnatural starches are broken down in the body, they release carbonic acid in the blood. In order to maintain the body's critical alkaline pH, the body pulls from its alkaline reserves, like calcium in the bones or magnesium out of the cells.

The sugars produced as by-products of starches are released more rapidly than the sugars that result from eating fruits. This inevitably leads to spikes in blood sugar. Excess sugars in the blood overburden the pancreas and eventually leads to the development of diabetes.

There are two types of diabetes, but in either case, the burden of excess sugar/acid in the blood and resulting overproduction of insulin makes the blood viscous, which causes vessel and organ

damage and chronic fatigue.

These same sugary foods begin their mischief in the mouth

by causing dental cavities. As we chew these foods, they leave

behind acid residues that eat away at the enamel of our teeth. And of

course, anything strong enough to drill through teeth, one of the

hardest parts of the human body, is most certainly capable of

dissolving organs like the pancreas.

Sugar Is a Drug

Although sugar is viewed as a food, it is technically a drug

because it produces a physiological effect on the body once

ingested. This is especially the case for HFCS. Like most drugs and

toxins, HFCS can only be metabolized in the liver. When the liver

metabolizes fructose, a cascade of negative effects go into play: A

by-product called uric acid is produced, which can cause gout and

hypertension; the liver becomes insulin resistant, dyslipidemia

occurs, and ultimately all these factors can lead to cirrhosis of the

liver.

Oddly enough, fructose is capable of creating the same illnesses as alcoholism. It can manipulate the same opioid pathways in the brain as heroin or morphine, which leads to the addictive behavior. Studies have shown that sugar can be up to eight times more addictive than cocaine. All of the markers for addictions to illicit drugs resemble the behaviors of sugar addiction. Physiologically, the ingestion of sugar leads to the release of opioids and dopamine, which produces the intoxicating sensation that ultimately carries the addiction.

Many studies have demonstrated that sugar stimulates the brain's pleasure and reward centers. These areas are located in the emotional centers of the brain. The dopamine release produces the 'feel good' vibe, and the opioids release produce the 'stoner-like' sensation. These same effects can be seen with nicotine, heroin, and alcohol. The consumption of sugar also produces cravings in its absence, bingeing in its presence, and withdrawals without prolonged usage, just like any other drug with addictive potential. The addiction is not an illusion, and the withdrawal symptoms can be just as painful as eliminating nicotine or caffeine. But this perfectly explains the sugar addiction, which has been nicely gift-wrapped as a harmless sweetener for pastries, candy, pasta, bread, ice cream, and cavity-laden drinks.

Here's an example of how this addiction turns into illness in our real lives:

How the Holidays Help Spread the Flu

During the winter months, it's common knowledge that patients are always the sickest. This is most often attributed to the change in weather that begins in early October and lasts until April. But let's examine how eating habits and culture play their part:

1. In late October, everyone gears up for Halloween by purchasing grocery carts full of candy to the tune of $2 billion in sales. Kids and adults alike return home with their sacks of 'white gold' and consume this acidic food for the next week or two.

2. Roughly three weeks later, everyone is sitting at the Thanksgiving dinner table, stuffing themselves as plump as the turkey with slices of ham, chunks of turkey, cranberry sauce, stuffing, green bean casserole, macaroni, potato salad, rice, yams, soft drinks, juices,

sweet tea, pies, cakes, cookies, and other goodies. Then that is followed up by seconds at the dinner table and take home plates. What is interesting is that the sleepy stupor and drunk-like state that ensues is often associated with the tryptophan in turkey, but it's actually our biology shunting blood from the limbs to the abdomen, sedating the brain into sleep to divert energy towards the digestion of all the acidic foods you just consumed.

3. No sooner than you're thankful for all the giving, Christmas arrives, and you're right back at it, with Christmas parties at work, the in-laws, your family, and then friends. With all the before mentioned foods, only now with several glasses of eggnog on top.

4. Once all the presents are exchanged, and the leftovers have run dry, New Year comes steaming around the corner. Glasses and bottles of high-calorie alcohol are poured on top of all of the mischievous nutritional behavior of the past three months.

Here's an epiphany that will knock your socks off: Why does the infamous flu season tend to rear its ugly head the same time every year? You got it! There's nothing special about the annual strains of flu bug (by the way, the predictions of which represent purely educated guesswork because the vaccines need to be created at least six months before every 'flu season'). No matter if it's bread, pies, cake, macaroni and cheese, potatoes, juice, or cranberry sauce, it's all processed sugar in the body that will create an acidic and toxic internal environment prime for infection and disease.

What is unique about the flu season is the impact of cold weather on our immunity, stress, and our holiday food choices. In a lowered immune state, the body becomes susceptible to everything from the common cold to cancer. The immune system isn't just our alarm system; it's an army designed to detect and eliminate any intruder that could compromise your health.

Sugar and Cancer

Our bodies are made of trillions of cells that are constantly being regenerated. Some of the cells end up going rogue and become cancerous. This isn't just for those who develop cancer; this holds true for everyone. Unbeknownst to you, your immune system has natural killer cells (NK cells) to stomp out these cancerous cells on a daily basis. These cancerous cells are marked for death, terminated, and then engulfed so that they can be eliminated from the body. When the immune system is compromised, these cells go undetected, and cancer growth eventually manifests itself as disease.

There are three key components that contribute to our immune system being compromised: toxicity, estradiol (1 of 32 estrogens), and sugar. All cancer cells, no matter where they accumulate in the body, are the same. They all eat sugar and excrete lactic acid. In the same way, lactic acid accumulates after vigorous exercise in the muscles; this lactic acid will eventually make the entire body acidic, creating a condition known as *metabolic acidosis*.

Here's where it gets dangerous. In an attempt to buffer the acid, the body will begin pulling from alkaline reserves again. The liver as a protective measure will start converting the lactic acid back into sugar (glucagon). And this is how the liver becomes a slave to the process of feeding cancer.

The evidence for this can be seen when we use positron emission tomography scans (PET). PET scans use radioactive tracers, typically in the form of glucose, to show the differences between healthy tissues and diseased tissues such as cancer. Of course, all tissues in the body are capable of absorbing glucose, but cancer cells use a much more significant amount of energy and thus more glucose when compared to healthy tissues.

Our ignorance of what is and isn't sugar is part of what's killing us. The saying what we don't know can't hurt us couldn't be farther from the truth. Sugar is so cleverly hidden behind the mask of 'healthy' that we're eating and drinking it by the barrels with reckless abandon. 'Fat-free' is now just a synonym for 'sugar heavy.' What they don't explain is, all that excess sugar will be converted into fat in the body. So think about that next time you're eating fat-free yogurt after a workout. One of the biggest lies ever told was 'sugar-free' drinks like Coke Zero. If you think a sugar-free drink is too good to be true, it's probably because it is. I'm not picking on Coke because, the truth is, the majority of other soda drinks are just as horrible. But Coke makes itself an easy target. They began promoting Diet Coke as a 'guilt-free' alternative in the 1980s. The drink didn't go over well with men because they associated the word 'diet' with being feminine. So, in 2005, they reinvented the drink and gave it the new name 'Coke Zero.'

Aspartame, the Hidden Poison

When we compare regular Coke to Coke Zero in relative terms, it seems to be a much healthier alternative. Regular Coke contains 44 grams of sugar, all derived from HFCS, and 140 empty calories totally devoid of nutrients. So the idea of a soda with no sugar and zero calories sounded like we finally could have our cake and eat it too. But what you don't know is, the Coca-Cola chemists have a secret sauce: the combination of two artificial sweeteners called aspartame and acesulfame potassium. All of the studies performed by the food industry have shown that aspartame is safe, whereas all *independent* studies have demonstrated that aspartame is a neurotoxin capable of increasing the risk for attention deficit disorders, Alzheimer's, autoimmune disorders, diabetes, and cancer.

Artificial sweeteners trigger the brain to produce intense sugar cravings that lead to overeating. This probably explains why refills are free at fast food restaurants and sodas are so cheap. What it doesn't explain is, why is there HFCS in the hamburger bun and ketchup? But who are we kidding at this point they've laced everything from baby formula to pasta sauce with added sugar to tantalize our taste buds. As you debate between which of the added sugars are the healthiest option—agave, stevia, or brown sugar—the truth remains:

There is no healthy version of added sugar.

Any sugar that has been extracted then adulterated can be detrimental to your overall well-being. No, you won't die by having a cube of sugar in your green tea, but Americans are consuming *twenty* teaspoons of added sugar on a daily basis. At some point, we have to accept that we don't have a sweet tooth; what we really have is a well-masked addiction.

The Antidote to Sugar Is Fiber

When sugar, especially fructose, is not consumed in its whole form, it can become a poison. This is why wherever you find fructose in nature, you will also find a significant amount of fiber. As Dr. Robert Lustig states in *The Bitter Truth About Sugar,* "When God made the poison, he packaged it with an antidote." That antidote is *fiber.* This is why when sugar is removed from fiber, it goes from being a harmless treat to a sheep in wolf's clothing. Fiber plays a critical role in slowly releasing natural sugars from plant-based foods, which lowers the need for insulin and makes you feel full. So whole natural fruits are never an issue, especially if they are in season and are seeded.

There are over fifty different alias names for added sugar hidden in unsuspecting foods like mayonnaise, bacon, bread, and granola. You would be hard-pressed to find any food not in the produce section of the grocery store that doesn't contain added sugar in some form. Below are some of the aliases sugar goes by:

45 Different Aliases of Added Sugar

Agave nectar	Maltose	Dextrose
Beet sugar	Fruit Concentrate	Sucrose
Blackstrap Molasses	High-Fructose Corn Syrup	Barley Malt
Buttered syrup	Rice Syrup	Cane juice crystals
Caramel	Castor sugar	Brown Sugar
Carob syrup	Coconut sugar	Confectioner's sugar
Date sugar	Evaporated cane sugar	Fruit juice
Golden sugar	Golden syrup	Grape sugar

Honey	Maple sugar molasses	Raw sugar
Turbinado sugar	Corn syrup	Dextrin
Glucose	Fructose	Maltodextrin
Lactose	D-ribose	Galactose
Corn syrup solids	Diastatic malt	Ethyl maltol
Brown rice syrup	Sucanat	Yellow sugar
Invert sugar	Treacle sugar	Muscovado sugar

Currently, the American Heart Association (AHA) recommends that men have no more than 9 teaspoons of added sugar daily (38 grams), women limit themselves to 6 teaspoons daily (25 grams), and children be restricted to 3–6 teaspoons (12–25 grams) daily. We're all consuming three times that amount, and in my opinion, even the recommendations made by the AHA are too much when you consider the addictive nature of added sugar and how sick we are.

You Don't Need to Be a Slave to Sugar!

One American family decided to conduct an experiment, with themselves as the guinea pigs, and go sugar-free for an entire year. The very idea of no added sugar for a day would cause most parents to scoff at the mentioning of it because of the potential backlash from the kids whining. But the Schaub's took on the task, and one year later, one of the most noticeable changes was their taste buds had completely changed. Their cravings for sugar had virtually disappeared. Fruits seemed to more than satisfy their sweet tooth and became their primary desserts. Their palates had become so sensitive to sugar that most of the sweet treats they previously enjoyed were now repulsive. Their entire family had more energy, got sick less, and the kids missed significantly fewer school days. My suggestion is to try it for 30 days. You'll be amazed!

6.

Seeds of Deception

Then God said, I give you every seed bearing plant on the face of the whole earth and every tree that has fruit with seed in it. They will be yours for food. —Genesis 1:29

There are seeds of deception carefully woven into the very same scientific community that has been deemed responsible for providing the public with information critical to health and well-being. For every study, peer-reviewed journal, expert opinion, or agency dismissing buying organic, going vegan, or boycotting genetically modified organisms (GMOs), there seems to be an equal number in opposition. It leaves us all confused and not knowing who to trust, so the majority of people end up aligning with what is comfortable and most palatable instead of doing the research for themselves and tapping into their own common sense.

The medical community, in particular, spends too much time philosophizing and defining diseases instead of determining the root cause of the affliction. So, despite being the pink elephant in the room, the cause progressively enlarges itself in the shadows.

Riddle me this: What is the use of defining why water is wet if you never take a sip and then die from dehydration?

Or better yet, what purpose does it serve to observe the progressive degeneration of a patient with diabetes as they lose a limb, go blind, have an ischemic stroke, compromise their kidney function to the point of dialysis, and then die of heart attack without ever recommending they remove the foods that caused the condition to begin with?

Our arrogance and willingness to maintain our blissful addiction to poor food choices makes us underestimate the true value of health and our magnificent ability to self-heal. Most of us maintain our bodies in the same way we maintain our cars, with the least amount of maintenance necessary. We would quickly change our entire perspective if we only knew half of the capabilities of the majestic machinery we call our body. Our skin is intelligent enough to determine the sensation of hot and cold without the necessity to actually touch anything; our middle ear can detect the body losing

equilibrium; objects can be picked up out of our peripheral vision

while maintaining our direct line of sight in order to perceive that

which we are not consciously aware of; our immune system can

immediately detect anything that is foreign to our body and quickly

mount a response.

And yet somehow we've lost the common sense to determine

what foods are poisons and which foods are nurturing.

No animal in nature is told what to eat. Not even a newborn

is confused about what its natural food is, as it begins suckling at the

onset of hunger when the mother is lactating, and her breast is near.

Maybe there is an innate instinct in infants that we lose as adults.

Infants and animals seem to understand that the food from nature

will provide nourishment, immune maturation, development of vital

organs, and aid in colonizing the intestinal tract with healthy

bacteria.

It's time we redefine food by removing bias opinion and

man-made contortions from the ingredient labels. True food comes

from and is grown alone in nature without the need for human

intervention. Once created, it never again needed God's divine hand because of its eternal growing cycle: a seed is fertilized by the earth, a sprout is formed, a tree grows toward the sun, the tree blossoms with fruit, the fruit ripens to be dispersed around the earth and eaten by living things, or falls to the ground to nourish the earth or animals who cannot climb.

The Invention of Hybrid Foods

The Industrial Revolution caused people to evolve away from what seemed to be a perfect sustainer of both man and animal. In the mid-1930s, people began mass producing hybrid fruits and plants. Today, more than 90% of the food available in supermarkets is hybrid in nature. These modern hybrid foods are higher in starch and fructose, which as I mentioned is several times sweeter than glucose and causes damage to both the liver and pancreas. This is why many of today's fruits are much sweeter than those grown in nature and have no seeds. The second generation of hybrid offspring are sterile and will not germinate. These hybrid foods are not consistent with nature's perpetual seed.

Here is a direct quote from Genesis 1:29: "Behold I have given you every herb bearing seed, which is upon the face of all the earth, and every tree, in the which is the fruit of the tree yielding

seed; to you it shall be for meat."

In plain language, this means that all of our food has been

provided in the form of herbs (plant-based foods) that come from a

seed and bear a seed; and every tree will produce fruit, and in that

fruit shall be a seed, and that fruit can be used for food. The word

'fruit' not only includes what we traditionally view as fruits but

ancient grains like quinoa, cucumbers, tomatoes, avocados, kale,

Swiss chard, and basil.

The vast majority of food sold by the food industry isn't food

at all but an experiment with nature's handiwork. The purpose of

this experiment was to aid farmers in producing crops on farmlands

on which natural foods would not grow. The inability to grow

naturally should have been a cautionary sign that this was not the

breakthrough idea it appeared to be.

Hybrid foods are created by cross-pollinating two different

species of plants. What is of importance to note is that 90% of these

hybrid foods do not naturally occur and will not grow without

human intervention and protection. Most are seedless and will not

reproduce in the second generation, have lower nutritional values, are extremely imbalanced in vitamin and mineral ratios, and their resultant sugars are not recognized by the digestive system, liver, or pancreas.

The wheat grain we eat today, for instance, was created by the same hybridization method in an attempt to produce larger crops so it could be farmed irrespective of its geographic region. The original grain was not starch based, but cross-breeding has changed the genetics of the plant.

In addition to the modification in genetics, hybrid plants become unnaturally high in starch and sugar. Starch of any kind is metabolized into carbonic acid in the body, which in excess can lead to an acidic biology that creates the perfect environment for disease to flourish.

The combination of starch with modified sugars produces a high glycemic spike that triggers the release of harmful blood concentrations of insulin. This deadly combo is a major risk factor for the development of heart disease and diabetes, which is why for diabetics, one of my first recommendations is to avoid certain starches and all hybrid fruits.

The sugars from starches are released by the liver much more rapidly than the sugars in green leafy vegetable and natural fruits. When these starches are cooked, the sugars become concentrated and become a major contributor towards obesity.

Hybrid Plants that Pose as Healthy but Are Hazardous

If you must consume starchy vegetables or grains, then consume them sparingly, uncooked or sprouted with a healthy fat like an avocado that will prolong the digestion of the sugars and reduce the glycemic spike. They should be used sparingly because these hybrid Franken-foods do not assimilate into the body completely and are stored as toxins, damaging the mucous membrane, and the sugars feed the fungus candida in your body. Some of these hybrid plants have been packaged and sold as nature's handiwork, but they are poor imitations of the natural healing foods originally designed by nature.

Some of the following foods on the list will shock you: seedless apples, seedless pineapples, seedless citrus fruit, seedless grapes and watermelon, beets, carrots, corn, certain potatoes, celery, broccoli, cauliflower, cashews, wheat grass, soy, aloe vera, white and brown rice, oats, several legumes, many bean varieties, echinacea, comfrey, garlic, ginseng, and goldenseal.

I can imagine you tossing this book at this point in frustration, so let me further explain why some of the listed hybrids that have been promoted as healthy are quite the opposite.

Rice

According to a 2012 report by *Consumer Reports,* rice eaten daily increases concentrations of *arsenic* in the body by 44%; a second bowl of rice increases it by 70%. These numbers were validated by FDA commissioner Margaret Hamburg. Over 60 rice products were examined. Some of the products contained five times the concentrations found in oatmeal and 1.5 times the Environmental Protection Agency's legal standard for drinking water. Brown rice typically contained 80% more inorganic arsenic (the harmful version) than its white counterpart.

Arsenic is introduced into the grains via the use of pesticides and poultry fertilizer. The chemical is absorbed on the outer shell of the grain, and because brown rice retains its outer shell, it retains a significantly higher concentration of arsenic.

Eating rice, which again is a starch, creates a chemical mixture of carbonic acid and arsenic. This chemical mixture produces a glycemic spike (dangerous for diabetics) and compromises the mucous membrane.

Corn

Modern corn, unlike ancient black corn, is one of the most hybridized plants in the world. The hybridized version depletes the soil of vital minerals and microorganisms, making the land impossible to be farmed in the future. Over 58% of the land in America is being used to produce crops like corn to feed livestock, which explains why the fertile Midwestern plains have been converted into a virtual dust bowl in less than 100 years. Today's Franken-corn is larger, sweeter, and more yellow and white compared to its ancient ancestor.

Garlic

Garlic is touted not only by natural healers; traditional medicine also commonly make recommendations for patients to use garlic. Garlic, however, is highly acidic. On the food chart, garlic registers at a whopping pH of 3.3, almost equivalent to battery acid. Due to an oxide allyl compound it contains, it weakens the cell and vessel membranes, which produces the artificial reduction in blood pressure. Not by any means will it kill you in small doses, but it's important to understand both the good and bad aspects of garlic's biochemistry.

Carrots

Carrots and carrot juice are often regarded as beneficial for eyesight. But in a society where the blind lead the blind, most health care practitioners are just as unhealthy and unknowledgeable as patients when it comes to nutritional medicine.

It is well known that carrots are highly starch based, but this undesirable trait is often overshadowed by its high concentration of beta-carotene. Beta-carotene is a potent antioxidant designed by nature to eliminate free radicals that lead to aging and cancer.

The modern carrot is a hybrid cross between Queen Anne's Lace and the wild yam. This vegetable was hybridized in Holland and should be eaten sparingly if at all.

The take-home point about hybrid foods is that commercialized hybrid foods create starch-based products that are imbalanced nutritionally. Although there have been foods that have hybridized through a natural process in nature, these foods were hybridized over the course of thousands of years, which allowed nature to make natural adjustments for adaptation. The hybrid foods being produced today are a knock-off version of nature's healing foods.

Soy

On the other hand, soy isn't necessarily a hybrid, but I could write a book on the dangers of soy alone. There's actually a great book that I suggest you read called *The Whole Soy Story*, by Kaayla T. Daniel. Soy products, like tempeh, tofu, and all meat and dairy mimicking products, often become the rebound lovers of those who abstain from meat.

Unfortunately, soy is a starch that produces sulfide in the body. This sulfide depletes the body of both iron and oxygen.

The brilliant scientist George Washington Carver was hired by Henry Ford to determine what uses could be derived from the soybean. In his genius, he was able to make rubber, ink, paint, glue, plastic, glass, and many other products. George Washington Carver, 'the father of the peanut,' was by profession a botanist and said the soybean should *not be eaten.*

Prior to the 1960s, not even ranchers would feed soybeans to their animals because it was well known to be a toxic plant.

Enter Dwayne Andreas in 1971 as the new CEO of Archer Daniels Midland (ADM), the American global food processing and commodities trading corporation. Andreas had made a name for himself previously at Cargill, related to vegetable oil. After teaming

up with ADM, he traveled the world in the 1970s and 1980s,

meeting with every major political leader from Castro to Gorbachev,

convincing them to adopt soybean oil as their primary oil of

consumption. His cunning persuasion and willingness to compensate

politicians who had parallel agendas earned him the nicknames

'Soybean King' and 'Deep Pockets.' By the 1990s, he had taken

soy, which was not considered safe for human consumption, and put

it in virtually every food product known to man. By the time he

retired, he had increased ADM soybean exports from $1.5 billion to

$7 billion.

Did I mention that 94% of all soy made in America is

genetically modified?

Genetically Modified Organisms (GMOs)

Beyond hybrids, what is of more cause for concern to the

health of the world's citizens and the earth itself are genetically

modified organisms (GMOs). GMOs foods are created through a

laboratory process in which genes are extracted from one species,

and through an artificial process, these genes are forced into a random position on the DNA sequence of an unrelated plant or animal. The offspring of this laboratory experiment is called a *transgenic organism.*

It's estimated that 70% of all processed foods today contain at least one GMO. An even more astounding factoid is, the SAD diet consists of roughly 69% of processed foods.

The majority of the tomatoes that Americans enjoy are the result of extracting a gene from the Arctic flounder fish that allows it to sustain freezing temperatures, and inserting that gene into a tomato which nature only allows to grow in summer. Now you can have tomatoes that can be easily grown during winter. If this appears to be an added advantage instead of a shocking undertaking, allow me to explain two things:

In nature, genes are only transferred to like species that can produce offspring and have similar genetic coding. In other words, in nature, a tomato and an Arctic flounder could never mate and reproduce. As a result of the random insertion and the newly formed transgenic species, the possibility for mutations becomes astronomical. These mutations result in the manifestation of disease, allergies, deformity, and many potentially harmful effects. Every single independent study conducted on the impact of genetically modified foods has concluded these transgenic foods damage organs, lead to infertility and immune system failure, and perforate the gastrointestinal tract.

The FDA's Cozy Relationship with Food Companies

During the first Bush Administration, the White House instructed the leadership at the FDA to create room for biotechnology food companies. So, in 1991, the attorney for Monsanto, Michael Taylor, was appointed the Deputy Commissioner for Policy at the FDA. Monsanto is the same chemical company that assured the general public that polychlorinated biphenyls (PCBs), Agent Orange, and DDT were safe, which we all know now couldn't be the furthest thing from the truth.

Once Michael Taylor was appointed, his role in implementing favorable GMO policy was done with a revolving door approach. He later went back to Monsanto, where he was promoted to vice president for public policy in 1998, before rotating back into the FDA and becoming the senior advisor to the FDA Commissioner in 2009.

In 2010, Mr. Taylor was named Deputy Commissioner for Foods at the FDA by the Obama Administration. He is the first individual to hold the position, which was created with a new Office of Foods in August 2009. I invite you to do a quick Google search on him referencing the FDA and Monsanto to verify this information. He is currently still in this position. The irony is that he was in charge of policy at the FDA when GMO policies were initiated and under the Obama administration, which made him 'King of All Things Food.' This occurred while the overwhelming consensus among scientist at the FDA considered GMOs to be dangerous and would lead to allergies, toxins, new diseases, and nutritional deficiencies. Unfortunately, all the research was met with backlash, and many of the scientists were fired and discredited.

From the first Bush administration up until the Obama administration, chemical companies that produce GM foods, including DuPont, Monsanto, Syngenta, Dow chemicals, and Bayer, have fought to suppress evidence, infiltrated our government agencies, and rewritten laws and policies regarding the food we eat that violate our constitutional rights. For this reason, it is almost impossible to pass legislation against GM foods because many of the government officials involved with creating and passing new legislation on food policy have become entangled in a web of conflicted interest.

The Suppression of the Pusztai Studies

These struggles have not been specific to America. In the early 1990s, Arpad Pusztai, Ph.D., a plant biochemist of Rowett Research Institute (the top nutritional research lab in the UK) was given three million euros by the UK government to determine the health benefits vs. risk of GM foods for human consumption. His findings and recommendations were to be used as protocols for all of Europe. He conducted experiments using lab mice, giving one group GM potato; another group received organic potatoes; and the third organic potatoes covered in Roundup Ready pesticide. Within ten days, the mice that consumed the GM potatoes experienced pre-cancerous cell growth, smaller brains, livers, and testicles, partial atrophy of the liver, and damaged immune systems. Only the mice group that ate the GM potatoes got sick.

Here is a direct quote from the study: "From the results, the conclusion seems inescapable that the present crude method of genetic modification has not delivered GM crops that are predictably safe and wholesome."

With the permission of his director, Pusztai then set up TV interviews to report his findings. For a few short days, he was celebrated, until there was a call from the pro-GMO prime minister to the director of the Rowett Institute. Pusztai, an author of 300 articles and 12 books, an expert in the field of botany and nutrition, and a 35-year career with Rowett Institute, was quickly fired, silenced with threats of a lawsuit, and his career smeared by the Rowett Institute, the UK government, and the biotech industry. It wasn't until his gag order was lifted by Parliament that he was allowed to publish his findings in *The Lancet* journal.

However, this set a precedent for scientists around the world for what would happen if their scientific findings contradicted the interests of the biotech industry.

In 1999, citing the lack of safety data associated with eating GM foods, molecular biologist Gilles-Eric Seralini co-founded the

Committee of Research and Independent Information on Genetic

Engineering (CRIIGEN).

Monsanto's Roundup

GM crops are sprayed with the chemically engineered

herbicide Roundup. The active ingredient in Roundup is glyphosate,

which was patented in 1970 as a broadband spectrum chelator. In

the soil, this chemical binds to many of the minerals needed by the

offending plant, preventing their absorption. It also destroys

microorganisms in the soil that provide nutrient to the plant and

promotes organisms that will kill natural plants. Since 2007,

Roundup herbicide is the most predominantly used herbicide in the

United States agricultural sector and second most in home and

gardening.

GM crops need to be genetically engineered to be tolerant to

Roundup. Most recently, in 2015, based on epidemiological studies,

the World Health Organization's International Agency for Research

on Cancer listed glyphosate as a category 2A carcinogenic in

humans. It's important to note that this chemical herbicide is absorbed into the foliage and transferred to the growing points of the plants, so merely washing the crops does not remove the herbicide.

Much of the livestock that is used for meat consumption is fed nutrient-deficient Roundup-ready crops, particularly soybeans and corn—neither of which is the natural food of a cow, chicken or pig. In the United States, factory farms raise 99% of all chicken, 99% of all turkeys, 97% of all hens, 95% of all pigs, and 78% of all cows that end up in the meat case at your local supermarket. These animals are treated brutally, stacked upon each other by the thousands, infested with disease, and grow so quickly that many are incapable of walking.

For those who aren't vegan or vegetarian, I would encourage you to watch documentaries like *Food, Inc., Forks Over Knives*, or *Food Matters* to get a first-hand view of what we're feeding ourselves and our children.

We can naturally assume that if the genes of plant and animals are being altered, *our* genes will also be altered as result of direct consumption of these Franken-foods because we really do become what we eat.

How GMO Foods Are Patented

Today GM foods are flooding American supermarkets. The USDA has approved corn, soybeans, tomatoes, potatoes, alfalfa, rice, papaya, beets, squash, apples, and many more. Most recently, the FDA slipped GM salmon into our food supply as the first animal product for consumption, without any extensive or peer-reviewed studies. This transgenic food, labeled AquAdvantage salmon, was created by taking the genes from the king salmon and using the promoter gene from an eel (ocean pout). The ocean pout grows and survives in freezing waters. The salmon, by contrast, typically stops reproducing during the colder months.

Unlike plants, Franken-animals *do not* require FDA approval!

Think about that for a moment.

You are the Food and Drug Administration, which functions solely for regulating and ensuring the food and drugs the public consumes are safe. Yet foods are being engineered in a lab and then doused with chemical pesticides, and the FDA has yet to require one human or animal study on the health effects of consuming these Franken-foods. Both the FDA and GM food companies like

Monsanto maintain that these foods are equivalent to naturally organic foods; however, the word 'modified' in genetically modified foods clearly indicates that these foods are not the same by definition. Furthermore, according to the FDA, nothing designed implicitly by nature, such as 'food' in this case, can be patented. No farmer could, for instance, pluck an apple from a tree and request a patent from the Patent Office. So companies like Monsanto, Bayer, Syngenta, Dow, and DuPont, which all by origin are chemical companies that now are in the business of making genetically modified foods, found a loophole to claim a copyright on their adaptation of nature's design.

On the one hand, these companies tell the FDA that GM foods are no different than conventional or organic crops and require no special testing.

At the same time, in order to receive a patent, they've convinced the U.S. Patent Office that GM foods are unique and nothing like natural plants.

Currently, the FDA's safety requirement for everyone on the farm table continuum is a self-monitoring program that encourages producers of new 'foods' and food ingredients to 'consult' with the

FDA when there is a question about an ingredient's regulatory status. The Plant Biotechnology Program, which was created in the 1990s, works directly with genetically engineered (GE) plant developers as a monitoring system, which is *completely voluntary* on the part of the GE plant developer. So the chemical companies themselves are legally obligated to monitor themselves and ensure the safety of food products they bring to the market.

All this information can be validated on the FDA's website.

Research Studies on GMO Foods

The Center for Science in the Public Interest, which has been a critic of food companies and their usage of unhealthy chemical ingredients, has not opposed GM foods on the grounds there is no evidence they are harmful. However, there are independent studies that show irrefutable data of the harmful effects of GM foods.

In 2012, the French published the first lifetime feeding study in the peer-reviewed journal *Food and Chemical Toxicology* that evaluated the health risks of genetically engineered foods. This study was conducted over a two-year period, which is the typical lifespan of mice. These animals were fed a diet of 11–33% GM

Roundup-tolerant corn cultivated both with and without Roundup

and Roundup alone (from 0.1 pp. in water; the level permitted in US

drinking water and GM crops).

The control group that was fed non-GMO corn had a death

rate of 20% for females and 30% for males as compared to the GM

corn fed mice that had a death rate of 70% for females and 50% in

males. Even the animals fed with low-dose portions of GM corn

died prematurely. The first females to die did so less than a year

after starting the GM corn diet and developed huge breast tumors.

The females at 21 months fed GM corn had a death rate that was six

times that of the control group.

Interestingly enough, the majority of tumors appeared after

18 months, well beyond the 90-day limit for food safety testing set

by the World Health Organization (WHO) and the FDA. The earliest

a tumor was discovered was at four months, again beyond the

standardized testing window.

Furthermore, the GMO-fed group experienced damage to

their organs and immune system.

When correlated to human years, we would expect these

detrimental effects to begin appearing as early as 18 years old, with the majority of the effects occurring around year thirty. Despite the fact that the origins of GMOs appeared in the early 1990s, we have only been consuming these products for roughly 16 years (far too long in my opinion). In that time, we've seen the same exponential increase in cancer and damage to organs in humans that was experienced during the long-term feeding study.

The World Health Organization has estimated that annual cancer cases will rise from 14 million in 2012 to 22 million within the next two decades.

Congress Sides with GMO Producers

Most recently, in 2015, the US House of Representatives passed legislation by a vote of 275-150 in favor of H.R. 1599, a bill that bans states and local authorities from labeling or regulating genetically engineered foods. The bill codifies a voluntary labeling system for the food industry but prohibits the FDA from ever implementing GMO labeling! It also allows food companies to make misleading claims such as 'all natural' for genetically engineered ingredients.

Public polls have consistently demonstrated that 9 out of 10 Americans want these products to be properly labeled if GMO ingredients are present. This is a blatant infringement on the rights of citizens, state, and local authority. American citizens deserve the same rights as the other 64 countries that require GMO labeling. The world's largest country by land area, Russia, created a national research project that determined that "As far as genetically modified organisms are concerned, we have made the decision not to use any GMOs in food productions," according to Prime Minister Arkady Dorkovich.

In Its Darkest Hour, Haiti Rejected Monsanto's GMO Foods

And if that wasn't enough proof, consider this: In 2010, the entire nation of Haiti was rocked by a catastrophic 7.0 magnitude earthquake. The nation was in complete devastation, with many of its citizens killed on impact and some still trapped beneath the rubble of collapsed buildings. They pleaded for help from every nation worldwide. In response, Monsanto sent 475 tons of GMO corn and vegetable seed. Although there were no laws regulating the use of GMOs in Haiti, the Ministry of Agriculture took a strong stance during one of the country's weakest moments and *rejected* Monsanto's donation.

Chavannes Jean-Baptiste, leader of a group of Haitian farmers called The Peasant Movement of Papay, referred to the donation as a 'new earthquake.'

In an interview, Jean-Baptiste said, "Fighting hybrid and GMO seeds is critical to saving our diversity and agriculture. We have the potential to make our lands produce enough to feed the whole population and even to export certain products. The policy we need for this to happen is food sovereignty, where the county has the right to define its own agricultural policies, to grow first for the family and then for the local market, to grow healthy food in a way which respects the environment and Mother Nature."

The farmers understood that if they accepted the seeds, they would no longer be able to reuse natural seeds that had been in the families for generations, the farmland would be ruined, and they would become lifelong servant-customers to Monsanto because only their seeds would grow there after using GMO crops. So, in a remarkable display of unity and protest, 10,000 Haitian farmers gathered to burn the 475 tons of GMO seeds sent by Monsanto.

7.

You Are What You Eat

Eat to live, not to Die. —Dr. Sebi (Alfredo Darrington Bowman)

This next concept is critically important to you understanding the connection between nutrition and disease. Once you are able to fully comprehend this, you'll become what I'd like to refer to as a 'conscious eater.' Each time you grab a bite to eat, you will be able to easily decipher whether the food is a producer of health, energy, healing or promoter of death.

So let's begin.

We must redefine what is 'food.' There are so many things that are passed off as food it makes shopping for real food a challenge. Walking into a modern supermarket gives you the notion that there are thousands of choices to consider for your dining pleasure. However, the produce section is the only section that would constitute 'true food,' and even many of those choices are quickly becoming questionable. So there is no such thing as 'junk food'; there's junk, and then there is food, simply put. Too many of us are eating with the purpose of satisfying our taste buds without ever considering food as fuel, nourisher, cleanser, healer, connection to nature, and the source of what you and I are made of.

The old adage "You are what you eat" is literally true, meaning the food you eat becomes the body you are made of. Metaphorically, once any non-living thing is created, such as a house, it does not grow; it has become its potential unless an external force such as yourself makes a modification. However, living things are not bound by this constraint. While we as humans may be born weighing just eight pounds, the body through divine sorcery uses nutrition to grow you into seven-foot, 325-pound Shaquille O'Neal.

The human body also has magical regenerative powers to replace the cells lining the stomach and colon every four or five days, the entire skin in 28 days, a large portion of your liver in six months, and your skeletal system every ten years. Your body generates the cells that become your new liver, skin, and bone directly from the foods you eat. Old cells die by a process known as 'apoptosis,' and new cells are generated from the foods you eat. So, if you eat processed, refined, genetically modified, hybrid, or Franken-foods, then it makes sense that you will become overweight, disease-ridden, and lethargic. Whereas if you eat vital live whole plant-based foods, you will be filled with youthful vigor and appearance and have an overall sense of well-being.

The Life Energy of Living Foods

Live foods transfer their life force energy into you as a result of eating and metabolizing them. This is simply the First Law of Thermodynamics in motion; energy is neither created nor destroyed but simply transferred. Dead animal flesh, processed, refined, hybrid, and genetically modified foods have little to no life force energy to transfer. In addition, these foods carry a toxic load that eventually stimulates and perpetuates disease.

New technology using Kirlian photography provides a unique visual of the unseen energy fields present in any organic material, such as plants. Kirlian technology uses 50,000 volts and a broad range of frequencies that transverse through biological systems (in this case foods) and magnifies the energy fields present, producing a visual image.

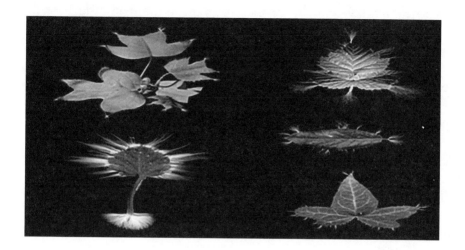

The light you see being emitted from these plants are biophotons, which contain essential information communicated from divine nature to transfer nutrition, intracellular consciousness, evolution, growth, and healing. The information is transferred wirelessly, like texting or calling from a cellphone, through thin air from the sun into the plants we eat.

This should be no surprise at all, considering all technology is based on nature, but these photos show why it's so critically important to eat *living foods*. Kirlian photographs demonstrate that raw organic foods display the highest energy levels versus the cooked and processed foods that give off a dull vibratory signature.

The Human Body is Electric

Our bodies run on electricity in the same fashion as any electrical appliance, using an electrochemical gradient of ions, such as the sodium/potassium pump, to synthesize ATP (energy). This energy is consistent with life, and we see, for example, when a patient's heart stops beating, medically we respond by using electricity via a defibrillator to reestablish a sinus rhythm in the heart. (It is referred to as a sinus rhythm because the electrical impulse originates at the sinus node located in the right atrium of the heart.) This electricity flows through your entire nervous system, sending electrical impulses to your brain to propagate thought, to your heart to produce a heartbeat, and down your spine and into your muscles to produce contraction and relaxation.

Your body does this very much like an alkaline battery. Much like the battery, we also use alkaline electrolytes to forge needed chemical reactions, but also to buffer acidic foods we eat. When the burden becomes too great because of prolonged neglect and abuse, we deplete our electrolyte/alkaline reserves, which sets the stage for disease to manifest itself in an acidic internal environment. Dr. Otto Warburg, winner of the 1931 Nobel Prize in physiology, stated, "No disease, including cancer, can exist in an alkaline environment, and every single person who has cancer has a pH that is too acidic."

Let's review how foods make an impact on biology.

You Are What You Eat—and Drink

Our brains are metabolically active for roughly 12 hours a day, and the brain is roughly 75% water. The primary method of removing metabolic waste from the brain is via proper hydration. Begin your day with water as soon as you rise; drink water before showers, prior to meals, during exercising, between meals, and before going to bed.

You should religiously avoid dehydrating foods and beverages like coffee, soda, caffeinated teas, sugary foods, and processed grains. Coffee also depletes the body of the 'happy molecule' serotonin, especially when taken on an empty stomach, which can lead to stress, anxiety, and depression. Our short-term decision of what we eat and drink can make us happy, but the consequences of those decisions can make us sad.

Outside of personal relationships, our most intimate connection is what we eat and drink. We crave it, we celebrate with it, it nourishes us, and it cures our loneliness when no one else is there. Plants respond in the same way to nourishment. It's been scientifically proven that when gardeners play soothing music or even talk to plants and say "I love you," they grow stronger.

Food is one of our primary methods of self-love. And how do we define 'love'? We define love as an incredibly powerful and passionate interest or pleasure in someone or something. It is not defined as an adjective but a verb and a state of being. So the proverbial question, "Do you love me?" can be more accurately assessed by simply observing one's actions.

The more important question is, "Do you love *yourself*?"

If so, are your actions and state of being in alignment with love?

Are your thoughts positive?

Are you eating and drinking foods to produce a healthy body and mind, or are you just feeding your desires to death?

Choosing to go with the status SAD diet is not an act of love. With every nutritional choice you make, whether it be conscious or subconscious, you are either making a choice to live or a choice to dig an early grave with your fork and knife.

These choices often have a physical and emotional foundation, but there is also a spiritual component.

Food and the Spirit

Our addiction to food and overeating is often an attempt to provide ourselves with self-love. In eastern cultures, this behavior can be traced back to an imbalance in one of our energy centers in the body called *chakras*. Overeating is often connected to the lowest energy system called the *root chakra*. This chakra is related to your physical body's need for survival, stability, and our relationship with our mother. The chakra is located at the base of your spine, and hence it's also referred to as the ground chakra. It establishes the deepest connection with your physical body, your surroundings, and the earth itself. Because of the deep connection to your physical body, it is also very much connected to your physical health. Its priorities are air, water, food, shelter, empowerment, and stability.

Poor nutritional habits send a subconscious message to your entire being that says, "You are not valuable enough to take the time

and effort to properly nourish your body with healthy foods."
Changing your relationship with food creates a sense of trust,
security, and connectedness between the mind and body. It tells the
body, "I respect you for housing my mind and soul in your sacred
temple." The body tells the mind, "I honor and trust you for spiritual
growth and survival."

Interestingly enough, your arms and hands, which extend
from your heart (love) chakra, manifest the physical love you create
in life, such as gardening, building a home, caressing a child,
painting a Picasso, or cooking. During the process of food
preparation, you are also infusing loving energy into the food via
your hands from your heart. This energy is transferred only from
one organic substance to another, and when living foods are eaten,
you receive a burst of energy from the exchange.

As Ann Wigmore, author of *The Hippocrates Diet and
Program*, so elegantly stated, "The food you eat can be either the
safest and most powerful form of medicine or the slowest form of
poison." Only foods powered by the sun and nurtured by earth are
capable of producing a healing effect on our bodies. So the reality of

today's society is that we are not eating real foods; we are ingesting processed and genetically modified foods sprayed with chemicals.

Beyond food choice, most people have forfeited all of their rights to self-heal and have handed over proper prevention in exchange for drugs. Our well-being has been put in the hands of healthcare professionals who have been educated and trained with the same philosophies of the very system that is poisoning us.

There's Profit in Chronic Illness

I'll be the first to say that 99% of healthcare professionals have your best interest at heart and have chosen their profession in an attempt to be caretakers of the sick and needy. However, the sad truth is that the textbooks, university studies, curriculum, drug trials, and continuing education are all funded in large majority by the same companies that profit off your misery and ignorance. Here's the sad truth: There is no money in curing diseases, but there's no money in dying a quick death either unless you're a mortician. The real money is snuggled right in between the two: the fat, sick, and nearly dead who live a poor extended quality of life propped up by therapies never designed to cure them of their actual ailment because they do not address the actual cause of the disease. True health can only be maintained and regained by prevention, and prevention's greatest weapon in the war on chronic disease, premature death, and compromised immune systems is live foods and waters, with adequate physical activity, and a sound mind and spirit.

The US Doesn't Have Healthcare; We Have Sickcare

As Americans, we've gotten so far away from living in accordance with natural law, the entire country's health is in shambles. In America, 20% of our gross domestic product (GDP) is consistently being allocated towards healthcare costs. Our expenditures towards healthcare, which is in the trillions, represents the entire GDP for many other countries. By comparison, France allocates 11.7%, Germany 11.3%, Japan 10.3%, Brazil 9.7%, and China only a mere 5.6 percent. Even more shocking is the fact that despite our supremely large investment in healthcare, our return on that investment has routinely ranked America globally around 37th, behind all of the before mentioned countries and every other developed nation. In 2014, the U.S ranked worst in healthcare in the developed world, while 16 other developed nations ranked higher.

So how is it that despite having access to the most advanced medical technology and drugs, Americans are the sickest and most morbidly obese people in the world? The valuable lesson to learn from this is health cannot be purchased even with the most advanced technology or the most expensive drugs. It is earned and given freely when you obey the natural laws that come with this sophisticated machinery we call the human body. And like any complicated machinery, the efficiency in which it operates is directly related to how closely the owner follows the set of instructions that came with the product.

Here's a great metaphor to compare how we treat our bodies versus the luxurious things we buy. If you purchase a Rolls Royce automobile, it comes with a maintenance package and operational instructions. You could retain the services of the best mechanical engineers and purchase additional fluids and replacement parts that are far beyond exceptional. However, if you decide that you want to fuel your Rolls Royce with liquid gold or jet fuel instead of the suggest premium gasoline, then you will have violated the manufacturer's instructions and would cause irreparable damage to your car.

This is what we do to our bodies when we decide to eat foods that were prepared in a lab instead of a garden. If you feed yourself, your children, and your family crap food, then you will look, feel, and have the health that crap food provides. The food designed for humans is organic, whole, living, and plant-based.

So, are we really what we eat? Of course, we are. Every day, 50 to 70 billion cells undergo a programmed cell death because every cell in the body has an intrinsic 'shelf life' set to expire at different times, depending on the type of cell it is.

Think of your body as a huge skyscraper that requires constant maintenance. If you eat the SAD diet, it's the equivalent of using cardboard boxes and duck tape as your building materials. Eating a plant-based, whole-foods diet would be like using bricks and mortar. What's even more fascinating about the concept of 'we are what we eat' is that when we make the switch to a plant-based lifestyle, the impact is almost instantaneous. We feel more energetic, less achy, no bloating, and have more clarity. No sooner than a week or two later, and you'll be receiving compliments about your glowing skin and vibrant mood. And before you know it, all the skeptics will be curious about what and how you're achieving such great health!

8.

H₂O: The Perfect Solution

It's time to rethink what you drink. —Dr. Bobby Price

Our planet is mostly covered by water, but not always where we need it.

Water covers roughly 75% of the surface of the earth. However, 97% is undrinkable because it is in the form of salt water. So only 3% of the world's most abundant resource is drinkable, and 77% of that water is frozen, of the remaining 23%, only half a percent is available to supply the needs of all terrestrial creatures and plants.

With statistics like that, you would think water would be a more precious commodity than gold, diamonds, or oil; yet with the twist of a faucet, we can take a carefree 30-minute shower.

Here's an even more interesting statistic: Like the earth's surface, our bodies are also composed roughly of 75% water.

You can begin to see why dehydration tightropes a delicate line between severe neglect and suicide. On average, we sweat out about two cups of water per day (without consideration for extremely hot weather or exercise, this would increase the depletion), we lose a little more than a cup via exhalation, we also eliminate six cups via defecation and urination. This is where the recommendation for 8–10 cups of water daily comes from.

In conjunction with this water lost, we also lose critical electrolytes and minerals such as magnesium, calcium, sodium, and potassium, which aid in the regulation of the body's fluids. These electrolytes are also key in neutralizing the acidic foods and beverages consumed, as I mentioned before.

The Many Problems of Dehydration

Being a chemist, I have a unique understanding and respect for the importance of having the right kind and amount of water. Researchers have concluded that up to 75% of Americans suffer from chronic dehydration. In 37% of Americans, the thirst mechanism has become so weak due to prolonged neglect; they fail to respond to the common signs of thirst like dry mouth, chapped lips, dry eyes, or ashy skin.

The symptoms of chronic dehydration are often mistaken for illnesses. Some of these misdiagnoses include:

Weight Gain

When the body's cells are depleted of water, they will then send out a signal alerting the mind of the body's need for water, which is often confused with *hunger*. This mistaken identity leads to increased caloric consumption. In addition, in a state of dehydration, the body will resist the urge to metabolize fat because of the absence of a safe medium to remove the toxins that are most often stored in fat cells. That is, if the body lacks a sufficient amount of water to neutralize the toxins that are stored in fat, the body will resist burning fat as a fuel.

Dermatological Issues

Did you know the skin is the largest organ system in the body? During chronic dehydration, the skin is the first organ system to be denied water. This leads to a reduced elimination of toxins and healthy oils, causing the pores to become packed with toxic waste, leading to acne, discoloration of the skin, chapped lips, premature wrinkling, bags under the eyes, dermatitis, psoriasis, and overall dryness of the skin.

Chronic Fatigue

Almost every bodily function requires water to take place. Even small imbalances in our hydration greatly affect our alertness. When we are dehydrated, our blood volume drops correspondingly. This causes the heart to pump harder in order to maintain blood pressure. This is critical because this pressure is what allows efficient circulation to deliver vital nutrients to the organs, muscles, and every cell in the body. Chronic dehydration will eventually redirect the blood away from the skin to the muscles and organs and impair your ability to diffuse heat, causing the core temperature to increase. This is what leads to rapid fatigue, muscle cramps, and light-headedness.

You can now see why simply resting will not cure you of chronic fatigue syndrome. Ensuring you are properly hydrated with water containing natural electrolytes is one of the best solutions to fatigue.

Depression

The brain contains roughly 75% water. During bouts of chronic dehydration, the brain's functions can become severely compromised. Dehydration depletes the body of essential amino acids that directly impact mood. The antioxidants tryptophan and tyrosinase produced in the liver are critical for brain function, but their production becomes compromised as a result of dehydration. The neurotransmitters serotonin, melatonin, indolamine, and tryptamine all function as part of the integrity of a balanced mind state, and all of these neurotransmitters are the by-products of the amino acid tryptophan.

Serotonin is known as the 'happy molecule.' Interestingly enough, the most commonly prescribed antidepressants are serotonin reuptake inhibitors (SSRIs), which increase the presence of serotonin in the synaptic region. The list includes Celexa, Lexapro, Prozac, Paxil, and Zoloft (Sertraline). Within the brain, the amino acid tryptophan is converted into serotonin. However, in order for this to take place, an adequate amount of water is required to transport tryptophan across the blood-brain barrier.

Sleep Deprivation

As mentioned in the previous section, dehydration thwarts the production of melatonin in the liver. Melatonin is the hormone that aids in the control of your sleep-wake cycles. Based on the body's own internal clock, the levels of melatonin are controlled. The levels rise during sleeping hours and then begin to gradually reduce themselves as dawn approaches.

Water provides the critical medium needed for this hormone to be produced. Stay hydrated and drink a cup of water before bed to get the internal engines running. This will allow you to improve your sleep hours.

Hypertension

Blood pressure is the arterial pressure that blood exerts on the systemic circulation as it traverses the 60,000-plus miles of vascular highways in your body. Although its measurement can vary, depending on multifactorial components, hypertension affects millions of people worldwide and is a primary risk factor for cardiovascular disease. During dehydration, the circulatory system will constrict to compensate for water loss and to maintain pressure.

The constriction of the arterial vessels will correlate with a rise in overall systemic pressure.

Because of the reduced fluid volume, the body will attempt to retain any remaining fluids to aid in the neutralization of toxins.

One of the most commonly prescribed treatments for hypertension is a diuretic (HCTZ). Diuretics work by simply increasing the patient's elimination of retained water, thus lowering the overall systemic pressure. But here's the catch: diuretics will never cure the patient, and in fact, it's a certainty that once you are prescribed a diuretic, your therapy will be continually escalated with other blood pressure medications at some point. It should also be noted that the retention of water is a protective mechanism that aids in protecting you from the toxic internal environment that created the condition initially. These diuretics, although helpful in some ways, do not address the cause, and they worsen the patient's dehydration.

Chronic Constipation

According to the Mayo Clinic, chronic constipation is infrequent bowel movements or difficult passage of stools that persists for several weeks or longer. This definition, although more accurate than most, does not help us understand when an infrequent problem becomes chronic. Nor does it inform the patient of the severity of the issue.

The truth is, your bowel movements are one of the greatest predictors of your overall health, and the number of bowel movements should be directly associated with the number of meals you eat. The shape, texture, odor, size, color, and buoyancy are direct indicators of your diet and gastrointestinal functionality. These features can provide clues related to the disease process.

Fecal matter is comprised of fiber, 75% water, both live and dead bacteria, dead cells, and mucus. The SAD diet is deficient in fiber, lacking in foods with digestive enzymes, and water deficient. These are key components that contribute to a healthy digestive system. Attempting to treat constipation with both prescription and over-the-counter laxatives only further complicates the issues because these medications lead to more severe dehydration. There are no shortcuts: just drink the perfect solution!

These are just a few of the side effects of chronic dehydration that mimic themselves as misdiagnosed illnesses. Being that our very existence is comprised of 75% water, it would appear rightly justified that our internal biology would initiate what appears to be an alarm system, alerting us to our dehydrated state. A body in a dehydrated state will immediately begin rationing its deficient water supply based on the hierarchy of the organ system.

The brain will take priority over all other systems; this is due to the fact the brain is 85% water, receives 20% of the body's blood supply, and is the master control center.

At this point, you might question, *why aren't the normal signs of thirst sufficient for the task: dry mouth, chapped lips, dry skin, dry eyes, dark urine, or the sensation of thirst itself?* As I said before, dry mouth is often a last ditch effort to alarm you of dehydration. After prolonged neglect, your thirst mechanism is eventually silenced.

Many people believe because they are drinking *any* beverage, it means they are hydrating themselves. This is a common misconception. There's an assumption that drinking coffee, teas, sodas, sports drinks, and juice drinks can serve as a comparable substitute for an already perfect solution. When in fact those beverages are actually dehydrating in nature. There are many beverages that are dehydrating, like sodas, coffee, caffeinated teas, and juices that contain massive calories and chemicals that cause toxic buildup. Water is the only sugar-free, zero-calorie beverage you can have.

Caffeine Is a Powerful Drug

With no offense to the Starbuckers of the world (I know how you feel about your morning's brew), Starbucks does a magical job in marketing and promotions. People line up in a 'Pied Piper' fashion to consume its tasty beverages.

According to a 2010 survey conducted by the National Coffee Association, 54% of Americans over the age of 18 drink coffee every day, drinking roughly three nine-ounce cups daily. A December 2012 report by the FDA titled "Caffeine Intake by the U.S. Population" stated the average amount of caffeine consumed in age groups 20–45 years old was roughly 300 mg per day per person.

For those of you unaware of why it seems to be impossible to start your day without a caffeinated beverage, or why kicking the habit of drinking those beverages often elicits withdrawal symptoms, it's because caffeine is considered a *drug*. It's classified as a central nervous system stimulant because of the temporary boost in energy and alertness. But like any drug, the abuse of its limitations can prove detrimental. A tablespoon or 10 grams of caffeine will kill you. Naturally extracted caffeine is separated from coffee beans when exposed to high temperatures. However, the majority of caffeine in soft drinks is produced synthetically in Chinese pharmaceutical plants. And now the American population's love for caffeinated coffees and teas has been partnered with caffeinated energy drinks.

Many are drinking them under the assumption of 'all things in moderation'; however, let's examine why this is not a philosophy to guide your health. In 2010, Sunkist orange soda had a disastrous miscalculation of caffeine label content. The label read 41 mg of caffeine per 12 ounce serving while the actual content was 240 mg, six times the amount of caffeine. That would be the equivalent of three Red Bulls or 16 ounces of strong coffee. As a result, 40,000 cases of hyper-caffeinated Sunkist were voluntarily recalled.

This explains why caffeine is so dangerous because it overstimulates the kidneys to produce a diuretic effect leading to dehydration. This why your thirst can never be quenched by these dehydrating caffeinated beverages. It's like attempting to fill a bucket that has a large hole at the bottom. This constant loss of fluids creates a severely dehydrated individual, and carbonated water is not capable of hydrating the body.

The sugars in soft drinks have been replaced with the synthetic neurotoxin aspartame (sold as NutraSweet, Equal, Spoonful, Equal Measure, etc.), as I mentioned in the previous chapter. This poison is concealed behind the promotion of zero calories; however, it's 180 times sweeter than natural sugar.

How Much Water Should You Drink?

The common recommendation is that you should drink 8–10 glasses of water daily. However, this one-size-fits-all prescription is a bit inaccurate. It does not account for strenuous exercise, hot and humid temperatures, medical conditions, or whether you are prone to sweating profusely. Two to three liters per day can be used as a baseline recommendation, but if you are involved in any activities that result in additional fluid loss, like exercise, you will need additional water to meet the demands of your body. Generally speaking, drinking half your body weight in ounces of natural spring water is a good measuring tool.

The Poor Quality of Our Public Water

A serious and often overlooked consideration is the quality of water we're drinking.

In the United States, tap water is the municipal water that comes out of the faucets. This water is treated harshly with chemicals and then pressured through aged piping right into your clean glass. So the only thing clean about a glass of tap water is the glass itself!

We should treat water as the elixir of life it is. Nothing on earth would exist without it. The Japanese researcher Dr. Masan Emoto conducted extensive research on water and how its properties changed when exposed to various stimuli, such as words, thoughts, and feelings. In similar experiments with plants exposed to positive thoughts, words, and feelings, these plants grew healthier and more vibrant. Both plants and water exposed to harsh behavior and conditions had just the opposite effect.

Another quality measurement is comparing water in lakes and rivers near metropolitan cities to water in isolated areas, closer to nature. Measuring the content of these waters, we see a vast difference in the amount of minerals and composition of pollutants.

Some of the minerals common to natural water sources include magnesium, which is essential to muscle movement, protein metabolism, heart function, and blood clotting, among other vital functions. The daily recommendation for magnesium is 1–1.2 grams daily. Magnesium is involved in over 300 bodily functions. So when we are deficient, it will show up in so many aspects of our health, including sleep.

Another essential mineral is calcium, which is critical to strong teeth and bones, regulating nerve transmission, blood clotting, and muscle contraction. Like magnesium, the daily recommendation is 1–1.2 grams daily.

Although sodium is often vilified, it occurs naturally due to underground salt deposits. It is often supplemented as a 'water softener' and for purification. Sodium is critical to the transportation of nutrients throughout the body and balancing fluid levels. Natural sodium in its organic form has a positive effect on blood pressure, contrary to the processed inorganic form that is in many processed foods.

Potassium functions to maintain a proper acid-alkaline pH and proper electrolyte balance in the blood. A deficiency leads to fatigue, increase in blood pressure, muscle weakness, cramping, and anxiety.

All of these essential minerals are combined to create alkaline reserves that maintain the body's alkaline pH of 7.35 through a buffering system. They are constantly being withdrawn to counterbalance the acidic foods and drinks you consume. Once these alkaline reserves are depleted, they will begin to withdraw these minerals from areas that you need them, such as the calcium in your teeth and bones.

Tap water is treated with chlorine to reduce the presence of parasites and attempt to make municipal water biologically safe during its storage and transit through water main lines, tanks, and plumbing. However, it also contains fluorine, which in chemistry is well known to be volatile and poisonous. People often add a filter in an attempt to remove the chlorine residue and improve the taste. But most filters do not protect against parasites (*cryptosporidium and giardia*), heavy metals such as lead that leach from the corrosion of outdated pipes (as we have seen in Flint, Michigan), antibiotics, and a host of other ghastly critters.

As I said, water is the elixir of life; so all forms of life pursue water with the same ferocity as we do, just with more ingenuity. That's how all the critters end up in our water supply. By the way, the parasite *Cryptosporidium* is a waterborne parasite that is shed in the feces after reproducing by the millions in the intestines of its host. This parasite can withstand temperature extremes and even survive direct exposure to pure chlorine bleach. No antibiotics or other medical treatments can remedy this vagrant. This is why using just a standard water filter doesn't do the job.

Finding Healthy, Living Water

The most common option is now bottled water, which is typically labeled as either purified or distilled.

Before I describe their differences, be sure to patronize only bottling companies that have ensured the plastic they use is free of bisphenol A (BPA). This is an industrial chemical that has been shown to seep into foods and beverages from plastic containers and leads to a host of health issues, including cancer, infertility, and birth defects.

Purified water is filtered water that is further cleansed and purified through an additional purification process, which is typically reverse osmosis, distillation, or deionization. The final product has higher purity than tap or filtered water. You're probably wondering, because of my previous statement, *is distilled water just purified water?* It can be confusing. However, purified water isn't always distilled water, depending on the process of purification used. Despite the fact that in the process of distillation and purification, water is exposed to higher temperatures than either reverse osmosis or deionization, the most important fact is, neither at conclusion will contain adequate amounts of minerals and trace elements for our biological needs.

They are considered *dead water*.

Dead water will eventually leach minerals from the body. So, essentially, bottled waters like Aquafina or Dasani are clean toilet water deficient in vital minerals.

The process of distillation, reverse osmosis (usually in an acidic medium), and deionization all eliminate minerals in the process. So, if those minerals are not added back organically, you are drinking dead water.

Natural mineral water, or waters labeled 'spring water,' must originate from an officially recognized source. However, spring water does not undergo a two-year intensive recognition and regulatory process and did not have to be bottled at the source until recently. Spring water is the statutory name for water acquired from a non-polluted ground source. In the UK, spring, tap, bottled, and filtered water can be chemically treated, while natural mineral water cannot. So, from a common sense standpoint, the source of water should be isolated from major cities, like areas in the Himalayas or Mount Fiji. These waters are naturally cleansed via the process of rain and supplemented with minerals and trace elements by filtering themselves through the earth.

Again, natural spring water should flow from a natural spring and be bottled at that source. Natural spring water is naturally alkaline with organic minerals from the earth, not alkalized with chemicals to raise the pH. Artesian spring water is obtained from a natural source but bottled off-site, then processed and purified.

Mineral water could be natural or artesian water.

Can you see the confusion that the water industry is presenting us with? What's probably more confusing is the whole alkaline pH focus these days.

The pH of most bottled water is highly acidic, and tap water most certainly is. However, it is not enough to simply purchase the bottled water with the highest pH above 7 to replenish your alkaline reserves. Check the labeling or call the company to determine the source and location in which the water was bottled.

What minerals if any are listed on the label?

Is the container BPA free?

Are they labeling this water as artesian, mineral, spring, distilled, purified, or deionized?

Are these natural electrolytes or synthetically added?

These are just a few questions that you should know about one of the most important nutritional and health decisions you make on a daily basis.

You should only ingest *live waters,* which come from a natural source and are unadulterated.

To expand your perspective on the topic, live waters are also present in fruits and vegetables that contribute to your hydration.

Fruits and vegetables, unlike other foods, come equipped with their own digestive enzymes that aid in their own digestion and prevent you from using alkaline reserves. This is another reason why eating plant-based and lightly preparing your food is so vital. High temperature from cooking denatures digestive enzymes, kills nutrients, and removes live waters.

When You Consume Water Matters Also

Lastly, *when y*ou drink water is also of great significance.

Drinking large amounts of any beverage during a meal violates the very nature of our digestive machinery. This is because when we eat, our stomach releases pH-sensitive digestive enzymes responsible for reducing our food into absorbable chyme. When we drink large amounts of fluids with our meals, these pH-sensitive digestive enzymes are neutralized and rendered ineffective. It's better to drink a large amount of water 10–15 minutes before eating a meal.

The great thing about water is, it passes straight into and out of an empty stomach. This lubricates the digestive tract in preparation for food digestion, prevents overeating, and bypasses the issue of digestive enzymes being neutralized. During the meal, you can drink a small amount to simply clear your throat as you eat. As a rule of thumb, you should allow two or three hours after a meal to drink a large amount of fluids. You should also drink one or two cups of water prior to sleep and immediately upon awakening. This will aid in the sleep process and jumpstart you in the morning.

9.

Digestive Rest

Man lives on one-fourth of what he eats, on the other three-quarters lives the physician. —Egyptian Proverb

Today chronic fatigue is so common that caffeinated coffee, espresso, tea, or some form of toxic energy drink is ingested almost on a prescription basis. A lot of people feel like their day doesn't get started until they're spiked up on caffeine or artificial sugar to deal with the groggy low energy state they're confronted with every morning.

Have you ever taken the opportunity to wonder why is it that after eight, sometimes ten, hours of sleep, you still wake up feeling lethargic, hung over, beat up, and as if you've been doing P90 x the whole time? It's so rare to meet someone naturally bursting with energy in the morning that most people are annoyed by them! But the value of having sustainable energy throughout the day is a priceless commodity. So the big question is, after all that rest, where does the energy go? Most people seem to be getting zero return on their rested investment.

So let's talk energy!

According to The First Law of Thermodynamics, energy is neither created nor destroyed but simply transferred. When we eat, the food must be absorbed and assimilated in order to be converted into energy.

America is without a doubt the most overfed nation in the world, so we should be bursting at the seams with boundless energy, but it's quite the contrary. Most people will sneer at anyone who has the energetic nature of a drill sergeant. So I guess the real question is, once our foods are digested, what happens to this overabundance of energy?

The body has a total of 11 systems: cardiovascular, central nervous, skeletal, muscular, reproductive, lymphatic, respiratory, integumentary, endocrine, excretory, and digestive.

Each of these systems is critically important to survival and requires its share of energy for functionality. So, if you had to guess which system requires the most energy expenditure, you would probably assume the cardiovascular system. After all, the heart beats about 100,000 times per day and about 35 million times per year and pumps 5.6 liters of blood through the entire body three times per minute over a distance of 12,000 miles in one day. That's four times the distance across the United States from coast to coast or the distance from where I lived in Japan to my home on the East Coast of the United States.

But you would be incorrect!

Maybe it's the respiratory system. Considering after only a few short minutes of not breathing, we would die, and from birth to death, it is an activity we must consistently do even in our slumber. We breathe 20,000 times per day without even noticing most of the breaths.

But you would be incorrect once again.

You probably believe that the muscular system is the only logical answer remaining. This option would seem even more logical due to the skeletal muscle's lack of automaticity and efficiency. However, the skeletal muscle actually burns very few calories on a per pound basis, especially at rest.

The real answer is your digestive system.

So allow me to explain the magnificence and delicate balance of the digestive system so that you will have a healthy respect for its engineering and an understanding of how we often violate this system, and in turn violate our health.

Your 'Second Brain'

The digestive system has a mind of its own, both literally and figuratively. It is often referred to as the 'second brain' or enteric nervous system (ENS) because, in very much the same way the brain transmits signals, responds to stimuli, and records experiences, the second brain does exactly the same. It uses many of the same neurotransmitters to propagate these actions. For instance, 95% of all serotonin, 'the happy molecule' that is often the target of many prescription drugs for the treatment of depression, is located and manufactured in the gut. In addition, dopamine, norepinephrine, and benzodiazepines, chemicals which are the biological blueprint for drugs like Valium and Xanax, are found in rich abundance in the gut.

The ENS is embedded within the gut wall and can operate both independently and in conjunction with the brain. There are over 100 million more neurons in the gut compared to the spinal cord, making the detection of harmful foreign invaders an easy feat. In the event that a pathogen should arrive, immune cells immediately begin secreting inflammatory histamines to call in the troops, simultaneously triggering diarrhea and vomiting to quickly expel the unwanted critters.

Eating processed dead foods laced with hormones, chemicals, and pathogens provides a breeding ground for them to wreak havoc on your digestive system. And because these foods lack their own digestive enzymes and fiber, they will not be metabolized, which will cause them to fester and rot in the bowels. This is how we contribute to our own demise by digging an early grave with our own forks and spoons. This process is known as *autointoxication*, no different than drinking yourself to death.

The Dangerous Buildup of Toxins

Our health is largely dependent on how well our bodies eliminate toxins. Constipation initiates disease because bowel waste will eventually rot and become toxic. The toxins from that waste will leach into our bloodstream. It doesn't matter if you eat a vegan or the SAD diet, the real testament to health is *elimination*. Our core body temperature is 98 degrees. So the food in our bellies is like food in a pot sitting in the middle of the street on a hot summer day. In just a few hours, the entire meal will be no good.

The carbohydrates will ferment, the proteins will rot and putrefy, and the fats and oils will become rancid. In the book *Toxemia Explained*, Dr. J. H. Tilden explains, "One of the first things to do to get rid of any so-called disease is to get rid of toxemia, for it is this state of the blood that makes disease possible. Disease is a crisis of toxemia, which means that toxins have accumulated in the blood beyond the toleration point, and the crisis, the so-called disease – call it a cold, flu, pneumonia, headache, or typhoid fever – is a vicarious elimination. Nature is endeavoring to rid the body of toxins. Any treatment that obstructs this effort at elimination baffles nature in her effort at self-curing."

So disease is the body becoming exhausted with toxic waste as a result of an inability to eliminate via proper elimination routes and nature's attempt to eliminate those wastes through an alternate channel.

Once these toxins accumulate, they begin to be absorbed across the bowel membrane into the bloodstream. They will begin circulating throughout the entire body and concentrating in the weakest tissues. If the toxins settle in the pancreas, then the disease will be diabetes; in joints, then rheumatoid arthritis; and if they settle in the blood itself, the patient could experience high blood pressure or septic blood. No matter where the toxins settle, they begin changing the cellular function and lead to degeneration in that tissue. As these cells begin to break down, so does the entire organ system. The heart begins to fail when toxins are concentrated in the cardiovascular tissues, the liver in cystic fibrosis, or the kidneys in end-stage renal disease. This is all the result of autointoxication and checked elimination.

The Six Paths of Eliminations

There are six primary elimination paths for toxins in the body:

1. Skin

The skin is the first line of defense to all things foreign, but it also works in conjunction with other organs of elimination to remove waste. Every toxin that is soluble in water can be eliminated via sweat. The common toxins that are eliminated through the pores are the metabolic products of rich foods like meat, dairy, and eggs. Quite often acne is a sign of accumulated toxins from these foods being pushed out of the skin.

2. Kidneys

Many of the same toxins will accumulate in the kidneys because they are responsible for filtering our entire blood supply. The kidneys are so essential to our biology that we have two, despite the fact that we could survive quite easily with just one. The kidneys not only filter our entire blood supply to remove toxic waste but also excrete excess fluids. The nephrons within the kidneys replenish essential nutrients and water back into the blood supply while retaining some toxins and excess fluid. The toxins and excess fluids are eventually eliminated in the form of urine by way of the bladder.

3. Lungs

The lungs also play a critical part in detoxifying our bodies. They remove toxic waste from the body in the form of gases. The most common example of this is the exchange of oxygen from the atmosphere and elimination of carbon dioxide when breathing. If our lungs didn't efficiently remove carbon dioxide from the body, it would lead to respiratory acidosis. Using deep diaphragmatic breathing techniques, you could remove toxins from air pollution or years of smoking.

Our bodies are constantly on the defense to cleanse and detox the body of chemicals that put our well-being in jeopardy. Case and point is, after a night of drinking alcohol, our bodies go into a state of emergency and purging. A chemical produced by the liver as a by-product of alcohol is what causes the alcoholic-like smell to be released from the lungs.

4. Phlegm and Mucus

The phlegm and mucus produced during a productive cough or a head cold is another method used to eliminate toxins or infections. Many of the toxic foods we eat are mucus-producing and so are eliminated from the body covered in mucus.

5. Lymphatic System

The lymphatic system is considered the garbage-collecting sewer system of human anatomy. The lymph fluid can only be moved by the skeletal pumping action of muscle movement (which is another reason being active is so critical), and this is why the lymph nodes are concentrated near the most active joints and folds of the body. The lymphatic system provides a janitorial service, collecting and removing extracellular fluid, intracellular waste, toxins, heavy metals, infection, and waste collected throughout the body.

6. Digestive System

The king of all kings as it relates to elimination is the digestive system. But how much digestion and elimination is actually taking place? Today 50% of Americans have less than one bowel movement daily despite eating three to four meals, not including snacks.

The medical definition for constipation is defined as fewer than three bowel movements per week.

Pardon the interruption, but let's take a dive into the common sense pool.

The digestive system functions to ingest the foods we eat, remove the molecular-sized nutrition for assimilation, and then discard the remaining byproducts of metabolism. This means that none of the chunks of food we eat cross the intestines, just the micro-sized good stuff. So when we are constipated, it's the equivalent of trying to flush a baby's diaper down the toilet. Our digestive plumbing gets obstructed and backed up with bowel waste.

The primary difference between plumbing and our biology is that our digestive tract is designed for filtering into the blood various nutritious substances across the tissues of the digestive system. Constipation causes normally safe foods to become toxic because it will eventually rot, putrefy, and ferment. The toxins will eventually leak across the mucous membrane into our bloodstream. This causes the blood supply to become septic and concentrated. As toxins begin settling in our weakest tissues, causing degeneration, at some point this toxic accumulation will begin presenting itself as what we define as 'disease.' Meanwhile, the self-inflicted assault continues with the average American stuffing his or her face with three or four meals daily, thereby eating thirty meals in a week's time on top of the impacted bowel waste accumulating.

Does the scenario sound eerily possible for most people you know?

Doesn't it seem borderline suicidal to have ingested thirty meals and only eliminate three?

Take a Look in the Toilet Bowl!

No matter the frequency of our bowel movements, each poo explains a lot about the foods we eat and how well our bodies break that food down. A trip to the bathroom to 'do number two' has become a taboo conversation despite the fact we all do it. But I want to encourage you to start taking a look at your poo before you flush because it could tell you a lot about your digestive health.

Undigested food like corn could be telling you the corn is GMO or you lack the enzymes necessary to digest corn.

Floating poo could be caused by eating too many fatty foods or eating gas-producing foods like beans.

Black tarry stools could be a sign of gastrointestinal bleeding.

If your poo looks like soft-serve ice cream from McDonald's, then you're probably lactose intolerant.

Poo pebbles are often the result of a lack of fiber.

And really foul smelling poo indicates a problem with digestion, leading to bowel waste rotting.

But in any case, if you lack regularity in your bowel movements, you are accumulating toxins. So the body, using its own intelligence, attempts to eliminate toxins via the tongue, skin, kidneys, armpits, feet, sinuses, and even the scalp once it has determined the plumbing of the colon is not properly functioning. And in response, we use anti-allergy tablets that stop the removal of mucus, antiperspirants blocking the removal of toxins from the lymph nodes in the armpits, and laxatives that dehydrate and actually add to the problem. Chronic constipation will then manifest itself as fatigue, migraine headaches, cardiovascular disease, and even autoimmune diseases.

Fiber

In addition to eating the wrong types of foods, we often eat them in improper combinations that lead to checked elimination.

One of the chief tools of prevention commonly missing from the SAD diet to remedy these potential ailments is *fiber*. The World

Health Organization recommends an upper limit of 40 grams of dietary fiber daily.

This is *twice the daily average intake in the United State*s.

Fiber is the indigestible portion found only in plant-based foods. The bowel's inability to digest fiber is what gives its utility in cleansing the digestive tract like a sweeping broom. Fiber also slows the release and absorption of sugars, helping to regulate our blood sugar for management and prevention of diabetes.

You have *soluble fiber*, which turns into a viscous gel in the stomach. This gel binds to fats to aid in the reduction of cholesterol, lowering the risk for heart disease.

Soluble fiber is also a major key to maintaining a healthy weight by giving the feeling of satiation without the addition of calories. It's often referred to as pectin, gums, or mucilage on labels. Great sources of soluble fiber can be found in fruits, vegetables, beans, lentils, and peas.

In contrast, *insoluble fiber* does not dissolve during digestion. It passes through the bowels in its original form, much like a sponge absorbing water and cleansing the bowels. It can be found in the skins and peels of many fruits and vegetables, seeds, nuts, and sprouted grains.

Insoluble fiber also aids in weight loss, promotes regular bowel movements, and prevents many of the bowel-related health maladies such as hemorrhoids and diverticulitis. Insoluble fiber is often referred to as cellulose or lignin.

Most fruits and vegetables contain both types of fibers in various combinations. Cereals, grains, and bran muffins are commonly suggested as dietary fiber; however, recent studies are proving that this may be yet another false narrative in the field of nutrition. It's important to note that despite the USDA's recommendation, there is no human requirement for grains. All of the nutrients and fiber in grains can be easily obtained from eating fruits and vegetables. Most people now know that any refined grain is unhealthy for your digestive system. The refining process removes the fiber-rich bran outer layer and nutrient-rich germ core that contains all of the antioxidants, vitamins, and healthy fats. This leaves behind only the high-calorie carbohydrate-rich endosperm, which without its partner in crime (fiber), leads to rapid spikes in blood sugar when ingested.

Many of today's grains such as wheat, rye, barley, and spelt contain gluten, a protein to which many people are sensitive. It is often suggested that people with celiac disease and serious autoimmune diseases avoid gluten because of allergenic nature; however, most people actually are sensitive to gluten, but their symptoms are less severe and may include bloating, indigestion, gas, and cramping. Wheat, in particular, is especially high in FODMAPS, a type of carbohydrate that produces gastric distress. Even in the case where grains are gluten-free, many unrefined organic grains will still contain anti-nutrients like phytic acid, gliadins, and lectins, which interfere with digestion and the absorption of nutrients. These anti-nutrients increase the permeability of the bowels and lead to leaky gut syndrome. This condition produces bloating, abdominal cramping, flatulence, fatigue, skin rashes, joint pain, new allergies, psychological conditions, and autoimmune diseases.

Oddly enough, many of these anti-nutrients can be found in the fiber-rich bran portion of the grains that is so often recommended. In some cases, these anti-nutrients can be counterbalanced via preparation methods such as soaking them in water the night prior, sprouting grains, and fermentation.

It's my recommendation that you eat vegetables, fruits, nuts, and seeds as your primary sources of dietary fiber. Chia seed, flaxseeds, almonds, Brussels sprouts, onions, root vegetables, and berries are just a shortlist of the many options you have to choose from. Notice that all my recommendations are fiber within *whole foods*. You cannot simply sprinkle synthetic Metamucil or Polyethylene glycol in a cup or in food to replace what nature so perfectly designed into the fabric of plant-based foods. They will not have the same medicinal effect on the gut. Whole foods are a perfect combination of nutrition and fiber to cleanse the bowels, which creates a tremendous amount of health. In populations all around the world, it has been demonstrated that those who eat a diet high in plant-based fiber live longer and maintain leaner body masses with a higher quality of life years.

Fiber is also an essential nutrient for creating a balanced and healthy intestinal microbiome. A plant-based soluble fiber called inulin acts as a nourishing prebiotic to healthy microflora. Despite being a soluble fiber, inulin is able to avoid the breakdown from acid in the stomach and small intestines, allowing it to be viable for downstream microflora in the colon.

In addition to promoting the growth of 'good' bacteria, inulin also leads to increased calcium absorption and boosts immunity. You can include inulin in your diet by eating onions, leeks, asparagus, dandelion, Jerusalem artichokes, burdock root, and chicory root to create a microbiome utopia flourishing with happy bacteria.

Your digestive ecosystem is comprised of over 100 trillion bacteria, viruses, fungi, and protozoa. There are over 500 species and three pounds of bacteria in your gut. If we were to examine cells in your body, we would find that only 10% of the cells we observed would be actually human cells; the rest are microorganisms or bacteria. So you can easily imagine how crucial it is to maintain the delicate balance between what is often referred to as 'good' and 'bad' bacteria. Disease is initiated when this balance becomes tilted in favor of the 'bad' microflora like yeasts, parasites, and bacteria, or if there is a deficiency in the 'good' guys like *lactobacillus* or *bifidobacteria*.

Fiber is the perfect solution for intestinal cleansing and hydration in the form of insoluble fiber, and soluble fiber provides fuel through a process of fermentation initiated by 'good' bacteria. A high-fiber diet creates a much more diverse microbiome, whereas a low-fiber diet laden with high caloric nutrient deficient foods promotes the growth of inflammatory bacteria and weight gain.

The Scourge of Antibiotics

One of the most destructive forces to the delicate balance in our gut is prescription antibiotics. Antibiotics non-selectively kill all types of gut bacteria, causing a negative imbalance in the intestinal flora. The overuse of these drugs leads to *antibiotic resistance*, which is becoming an emerging issue in healthcare. Numerous studies have shown that concomitant use of antibiotics with probiotics during therapy and continued after the therapy helps to reestablish the microbiome.

Yogurt is commonly recommended as a probiotic supplement. Yogurt, however, is a sugary junk food that does more damage than good. Most contain upwards of 30 grams of sugar per container, and the amount of actual probiotic is sub-therapeutic.

The only milk product that provides intestinal health for humans is breast milk. It has been proven scientifically that the protective effects of the mother's own immunity can be passed on to the child via breastfeeding.

The most prudent source of probiotics will always be plant-based foods but if supplementation is necessary, then use a natural soil-based probiotic that has concentrations in the magnitude of 50 billion CFUs per serving.

Another tool to put in your arsenal to create great digestive health is properly combining your foods. Proper food combining was introduced by Dr. John Tilden and Dr. William Hay, and then continued by Dr. Herbert Shelton, all working under the premise that improper food combinations produced an acidic environment as a result of failed digestion and metabolism of these foods. This is what ultimately leads to constipation, depleted alkaline reserves, and toxic accumulation, which sets the stage for disease.

These improper combinations present themselves as flatulence, nausea, acid reflux, gas, constipation, and even malnutrition.

The Digestive Process

Observing animals in nature, we notice that they eat a single food type or in very minimal combinations. Eating our foods in either singular or minimal combinations aligns with our digestive biochemistry related to pH-sensitive digestive juices and enzymes. We use these digestive juices and enzymes to break down food into a liquid form so that it can then be metabolized into its nourishing components (macro and micronutrients, and enzymes). Thus, proteins become amino acids, carbohydrates are separated into simple sugars, fats are metabolized into fatty acids, and micronutrients are extracted into vitamins, minerals, and trace elements. Once in liquid form, they can be absorbed across the intestinal membrane into the blood, while the remaining by-products are eliminated from the body.

The digestive process occurs in three sequential stages, each requiring various enzymes:

1. In the Mouth

The process begins mechanically in the mouth, via chewing and the activation of the enzyme salivary amylase. This enzyme can only be effective if food is chewed for a long enough period to break down food mechanically. Salivary amylase in the mouth will break down only carbohydrates; it cannot digest proteins or fats. Proteins and fats must move into the stomach for digestion.

2. In the Stomach

The foods that primarily break down in the stomach are proteins, where both the highly acidic enzyme pepsin and hydrochloric acid are present. Contrary to popular belief, hydrochloric acid alone does not break down proteins; it provides the acidic medium for pepsin to do so with the assistance of gastric juices.

Starches are a form of carbohydrate that requires an alkaline medium for digestion, contrary to proteins. Proteins like steak, for instance, will require an acidic medium. This is why combining proteins with starches (steak and potatoes) during meals will cause the pH in the stomach to become neutralized, severely compromising the digestion of that meal. Once the acid-base ratio is compromised, the stomach, in an attempt to liquefy the meal, will overcompensate by secreting more hydrochloric acid and more pepsin, often leading to acid reflux and heartburn conditions. This prolongs the digestion time from what would typically be three hours to up to 13 hours in the stomach.

3. In the Small Intestine

The food then moves into the small intestine undigested, and hence not conducive to absorption. Any foods that go undigested cannot be used for nourishment, and thus will begin to putrefy and ferment, releasing toxins into the tissue. Hence the nourishment we receive from food is not dependent on *what* we consume, more so than how efficient we can *digest and assimilate* those foods. If the enzyme pepsin is neutralized by the presence of starches, it will fail to reduce protein foods into peptones in the stomach, and erepsin will fail to further reduce the peptones into their absorbable component amino acids.

For this reason, proteins and starches (whether plant- or animal-based) should never be consumed during the same meal.

I highly recommend eating starches very sparingly because of the acidic nature of these foods. You should wait two hours to consume any proteins after eating a starch or three hours to eat any starches post eating proteins. When properly digested, carbohydrates like fruits are reduced down to simple sugars that are quickly converted into energy and used as nutrients. However, when carbohydrates are improperly digested, they will putrefy and ferment, leading to the production of carbon dioxide, lactic acid, acetic acid, and alcohol. These compounds create an acidic environment that sets the stage for disease. For this reason, fruits should be eaten under a totally separate guideline. They spend a minimal time in the stomach, where they are only mechanically broken down then quickly passed into the small intestines where they are then chemically digested. Because of this quick and efficient process, fruits should be consumed alone on an empty stomach, or thirty minutes before eating any other foods. Melons specifically should be consumed separately from all foods, including other fruits. Fruit vegetables such as avocados and tomatoes are fine to eat with green vegetables, despite being labeled as fruits.

In addition to stomach gastric juices for digestion, we also produce the enzyme lipase, which catalyzes the breakdown of fats into fatty acids, and the proteolytic enzyme rennin, which curdles or coagulates milk in the stomach. Once a child has a full set of teeth, the enzyme renin is typically totally diminished, and there is no nutritional need for milk at this point.

As I mentioned in a previous chapter, dairy products are the equivalent of Elmer's glue for the digestive tract and lead to many of the allergic symptoms we experience; so it is my recommendation that you avoid all forms of dairy.

Following these few simple principles can create a tremendous boost to your health. As you can see, eating the most nutritious foods but failing to eat them properly can lead to nutritional deficiencies and toxic accumulation. Eating foods in proper combinations or mono meals is an excellent way to work *with* your gastrointestinal system instead of *against* it.

Therapeutic Fasting

My final recommendation that can be used for digestive restoration is *therapeutic fasting*. For thousands of years, this ancient practice has been used to rejuvenate, heal, and cure the body. Inscribed on a pyramid wall in Egypt almost 6,000 years ago is the quote, "Man lives on one-quarter of what he eats. On the other three-quarters lives his doctor." Ancient knowledge seems to stand the test of time, as America has become the most obese nation in the history of man. The Western diet, which is no longer exclusive to

America, is on its way to invading even the most rural countries around the world, creating an obsession for calorie-rich, nutrient-poor fast foods. The Western diet is a protein heavy, chemical laden, sugar intensive, refined carbohydrate recipe for creating herds of overfed and malnourished ticking time bombs.

A National Health survey found that 60% of adults and 30% of all children in America are either overweight or obese. America is just a microcosm of what is to come to those countries adopting the 'eat to die' lifestyle in all parts of the world. At its foundation, the typical Western diet or SAD diet is about 60–70% processed foods, which means 70% of what Americans consume is laced with chemical additives, preservatives, synthetic sugars, and many other uninvited biochemical terrorists. In addition, most of the nutrients in these foods are refined out through the process of food manufacturing. There is no section of the traditional supermarket that does not have food laced with chemicals. The aisles are stacked high with pseudo-foods poisoned with fillers, additives, food dyes, flavorings, stabilizers, and preservatives. Even much of the produce is riddled with harmful pesticides and chemicals. As the liver and kidneys become so oversaturated with eliminating these chemicals, in an attempt to preserve the integrity of the blood, these toxins are stored in the tissues.

When we eat processed and fast foods, we lose our ability to feel satiated, so we just keep eating. This is a cue that our taste buds and the sensation of hunger have been hijacked.

The perfect response is to *stop eating* and allow the body to recalibrate.

Now I understand that the thought of missing even a single meal brings a certain amount of anxiety, but I can assure you that once you begin to abstain from food, you will begin to heal. Fasting while consuming liters of natural spring water acts as a hot shower to cleanse the tissues on a deep cellular level.

In a satiated state, the body uses primarily glucose and fat extracted from foods as its primary energy sources. The pancreas releases insulin into the blood to facilitate the passage of glucose into both the muscle and brain tissues to be used as energy. Any excess glucose will be transported to, and then stored in, the liver as glycogen.

Twenty-four hours after initiating a water fast, these glycogen stores will be depleted. All the energy that is normally required for digestion is then diverted from manufacturing and secreting digestive enzymes, production of stomach acid and bile, the physical breakdown of food, water sequestered into the intestines, the peristalsis of the intestinal wall, and many other processes. All of this unused energy now will be diverted towards healing and restoration. As a result of an evolutionary adaptation during times of famine, our bodies are designed to fast. Fasting to heal is an organic process and can be witnessed in the wild or with domestic pets when they are ill. Most dogs will refuse to eat and go into a state of dormant activity when they are sick or injured.

The Healing Crisis

When most people fast, they often quit before they obtain any actual therapeutic benefits because they feel as if their body is having a negative reaction to not having food. What we often view as the body's adverse reaction to fasting is actually a *healing crisis* taking place.

A healing crisis, also known as a Herxheimer Reaction, occurs during a fast when the body attempts to eliminate toxins more rapidly than the elimination channels can remove them. These reactions occur as a result of the rapid detox of cells that release toxins, dead pathogenic organisms as a result of increased immune response and fever (high body temperatures help to kill pathogens), and endotoxins released from those microbes into the bloodstream that produce headaches, dizziness, fatigue, fever, nausea, and temporary infections.

During the first 24 to 48 hours of the fast, your body metabolizes glucose circulating in the blood and stored in the liver and muscle tissues as glycogen. These glycogen stores are depleted after the first 24 hours; however, the liver synthesizes new glucose from amino acids to maintain a normal blood glucose level during fasting. So the detoxification at the cellular level does not actually begin until the blood sugars are fully metabolized 72 hours into the fast.

My First Water Fast, Day by Day

In my own personal journey, days 1 and 2 were simply uncomfortable, and to be honest, it just felt foreign not placing solid food in my mouth. We're so used to having food part of our social construct that removing it puts us in an uncomfortable space.

But it's only when we enter these uncomfortable spaces in life that we allow ourselves to break routine and stretch our limits beyond our comfortable self-imposed barriers.

Day 3 of my first fast felt like I was confronting every myth I had learned about food and healing. Fatigue set in that made normal activity appear rigorous, and migraine ensued from all of the ingested toxins that were now circulating in my blood. I started to experience nausea from the layers of gunk becoming un-plastered from the lining of my stomach and now was stewing around in my stomach, and then a little dizziness from all of the above as my brain attempted to maintain its homeostasis in an acutely polluted environment. Yes, Day 3 for me definitely was rough, but I've also witnessed others experience none of these symptoms, so each experience will be patient specific. But at the time, I was certain I was approaching starvation. My cravings for sugar and salt seemed to scream at me minute by the minute. These were all withdrawal symptoms unrecognizable to me because I had never associated food with addiction. The entire experience at that point was new territory for me.

Between days 3 and 4, low insulin levels stimulate your body to switch to burning stored fats as the primary fuel. Fat, especially visceral or omentum fat ('belly fat'), acts as an organ of its own, retaining many of the toxins we ingest and releasing harmful hormones that cultivate disease. This, along with many other factors, can prolong healing, depending on the amount of fat and chemicals specific to the patient.

The stored form of fat is known as *triglycerides* and consists of a glycerol backbone and three fatty acid chains. Both the glycerol backbone and the fatty acid chains can be used directly and indirectly as energy in a variety of tissues, with the exception of the brain. However, fatty acids can be converted into what is known as ketone bodies in the liver, which are capable of crossing the blood-brain barrier to be used as energy. The release of ketones into the blood circulation suppresses appetite, which is a blessing from the heavens if you're fasting.

This is why by days 4 and 5, my body seemed to go into fasting cruise control. I began to experience an increase in energy, lightness, and an overall feeling of well-being that I probably haven't experienced since I was a teenager.

You will probably find it even more difficult to believe that despite having periodic cravings, which most likely could be attributed to pathogens like yeast remaining in the body, you most likely will not actually feel hungry at this point.

My first water fast lasted twenty-one amazing days. I lost 17 pounds and gained a tremendous amount of health in the process. The aches and pains in my lower back and joints went away, my belly bulge disappeared, I had a nagging knee injury that suddenly healed itself, I seemed to be more energetic at the gym, and my blood pressure was normalized. I've seen thousands of prescriptions to treat hypertension and have seen some patients on a regimen of four or more medications to 'treat' their blood pressure. I've never in my professional career, not even once, seen one patient cured with traditional medicine alone. I was initially just curious about fasting, but at this point, it had my full attention and helped me see first-hand the body's unlimited ability to heal when we remove toxicity from our body.

Having a first-hand experience with fasting most importantly made me question our approach to healing in modern medicine. I can't begin to tell you how humbling it is to have an education in the field of medicine valued at over $200,000 and realize much of what I was taught needed to be unlearned. That 21 days of fasting stands as one of my greatest accomplishments in life. But as beautiful as the experience was for me, I am not suggesting everyone just go cold turkey and water fast for 21 days. I was a lunatic in search of ways to heal the body naturally so that I could first heal myself and then show others how to take a more holistic approach to well-being.

Your First Water Fast

In general, I recommend that you fast no longer than 72 hours for your first fast, and you should consult with your primary physician to request supervision throughout the process, especially with a water-only fast. A water-only fast could potentially increase the blood concentrations of many drugs, supplements, and vitamins to dangerous levels, which could lead to injury or exacerbation of known or unknown conditions. This is critically important because some drugs cannot be abruptly discontinued; they require that you be weaned off over the course of time.

If your physician does not agree, and you still feel inclined to use fasting as a source of healing, then exercise your civil liberties and find a capable and willing physician or healthcare practitioner willing to guide you. A holistic approach can often clash with traditional medicine, but I can assure you there are a plethora of practitioners who are skilled and enthusiastic about your choice to choose a natural path.

If you are on medications that cannot be abruptly discontinued, or you simply don't feel comfortable with a water fast, my alternative suggestion is doing a juice fast.

Let me answer your question quickly before you ask it. Concentrated juices you typically purchase in the store are *not living juices*. If the expiration date is longer than a week, it will not serve you. I understand we live in an 'on the go' society, but if you don't make the time to use your own juicer, and you choose the more convenient route of purchasing them, then be sure to buy freshly cold-pressed juices that are not from concentrate and have no additives other than the juices from whole foods. If you check out the documentary *Fat, Sick, and Nearly Dead*, you can witness the challenges, benefits, and evolution of ordinary people like you and myself who were healed by juice fasting.

It is also important to note that consecutive day fasting is by far the most effective. But there are alternatives such as mono-fasting, alternate day fasting, and intermittent fasting, which do provide some benefit and I recommend for certain patients.

After your fast is completed, your body has to be gradually reintroduced back to solid foods. The beauty of this process is that now that you have experienced this level of detoxification, you'll be able to feel your foods more. I once went dairy-free prior to both my fast and introduction to veganism for 60 days and then made the foolish mistake of breaking the dairy fast with a slice of pizza. In short, I experienced what felt like the initial signs of a heart attack: shortness of breath, light-headedness, racing heartbeat, and blurred vision. So please don't make that foolish mistake I did by indulging myself in rich processed foods right after a fast.

You should first continue the juices and add small chunks of seasonal fruit. Next, you can add raw vegetables and soups. You can then slightly increase the fiber content of your meals with steamed vegetables and whole grains like quinoa, nuts, and seeds. This is an excellent way to transition into a whole-food, plant-based vegan diet. By this time, you'll be so excited about eating solid foods again that you will have a newfound appreciation for simple unadulterated whole fruits and vegetables. Your taste buds will have undergone an organic reboot and reset themselves back to their default settings.

This chapter on 'Digestive Rest' is like a pot of gold; reading this chapter alone could save your life and produce a tremendous amount of health. The world is overfed on processed pseudo-foods and starved into malnutrition from a lack of plant-based whole foods.

As I mentioned in Chapter 1, in Japan, there is an old saying, "Hara Hachi Bu," which means "Eat only 80%," or in other words, *never* eat until you're completely full. We are so used to overindulging ourselves with food we often eat until we feel sick. The reason "Hara Hachi Bu" makes biological sense is because our brains are several minutes behind our stomachs, and as a result, when we eat to 80%, we are actually full. The Okinawans, in particular, have embraced this philosophy and enjoy a higher quality of health.

You and the people you love can enjoy the same benefits by adopting these simple techniques that won't cost you the arm or leg that diabetes makes you pay.

10.

Going Green

Fruits for electricity, vegetables for grounding, herbs for healing, nuts and seeds for building. —Dr. Sebi (Alfredo Darrington Bowman)

When it comes to adopting a plant-based lifestyle as a solution to health and healing, I am certain that this lifestyle has general application to someone just like you. Because I am someone just like you, with the same range of human emotions, with similar strengths and weaknesses, and the same previous desire to eat meaty, cheesy, salty, fatty, nutrient-deprived foods.

I grew up eating the same traditional Western foods, and I had the same apprehensions and attachments to animal-based products for the majority of my life based on societal myths and family habituation.

I say 'lifestyle' as opposed to 'diet' because diets are trendy and unsustainable. They do not prevent, reverse, or eliminate any disease, as opposed to a whole foods plant-based vegan lifestyle. Dieting always ends with the dieter gaining back all of the weight they lost, and 67% end up gaining additional pounds. On the short list of diet fads are Atkins, South Beach, Jenny Craig, Weight Watchers, Zone diet, Blood Type diet, and DASH diet; all have epically failed among others. And now the scientifically unsupported Paleo diet is the new kid on the block, boasting itself as the new savior and the original diet of man.

I won't commit too many words to paper to address how off-the-mark the idea of mimicking our caveman ancestors is, but I will tell you there is no 'DIEt' capable of being a solution to health, wealth loss, disease, our environment, and animal cruelty. But the lifestyle I'm suggesting provides of all of these benefits plus more.

We need to radically change our prioritization to a 'health is wealth' mentality and 'food is medicine' approach because the foods we eat can either give us an abundance of life or a disease-ridden premature death. And contrary to popular belief, going plant-based isn't the extreme decision it's so often made to be; it's a return to our natural origins. The concept of veganism appears to be the new fad, but it's not a new concept at all. Scientists have discovered ancient Egyptians were predominantly vegan, as well as a long list of well-known historical figures, including Plato and Pythagoras of Greece, Leonardo Di Vinci, Benjamin Franklin, and Albert Einstein. Not a bad list to be on. In addition, people like Bill Clinton, R&B singer Usher, Woody Harrelson, Mike Tyson, Russell Simmons 'The Happy Vegan,' Stevie Wonder, Serena and Venus Williams during tournament play, weightlifting Olympic gold medalist Kendrick Farris, UFC champion fighter Nick Diaz, Mr. Universe Barny du Plessis, and now superstar Beyoncé is encouraging us all to follow suit. The list is long and debunks every myth about the necessity of animal protein for longevity, fitness, health, and beauty.

This lifestyle isn't just taking a small step away from the SAD diet, like many of the recommendations made in the traditional health arena.

It's like getting wings to fly.

Plant-based whole foods improve the quality of your life, the longevity of your life, and the world around you. These are just a few of the amazing benefits that new studies have confirmed. Even a small transition from vegetarian to vegan can show huge rewards by simply ditching dairy.

But being vegetarian, and for that matter just simply vegan, isn't sufficient, because these labels say much more about what you *don't* eat and less about what you *do*. Oreos and Doritos are vegan, but I can assure you they're just as bad as the other processed cookies and chips. I'm not suggesting that you eat tasteless food; I'm simply stressing the importance of ensuring your food be plant-based at its foundation and its cornerstone be vegan.

Now I know what you're thinking—*The last thing I want to become is a tree-hugging meat-hating vegan.* Vegans often get a bad rap for being labeled as judgmental, attacking, conceited, and just downright annoying.

Allow me to be the first to agree with you that some of us are. Some annoy the hell out of me. But it's often from a place of love. It's not an attempt to belittle you or back you down into a basement of shame, but it's a cry out to love yourself, animals, and the earth. To me, it's absolutely amazing how such a simple decision of what we choose to put at the other end of our fork becomes such a powerful choice. It's not only capable of changing your life, but it's also powerful enough to save it, and even the life of another animal. Because every time you eat a plant-based burger instead of beef, chicken, pork, or fish, you're voting with your dollars.

I wrote this book to empower you to take your health back into your own hands.

We are far more powerful than we know.

When laws and policies are passed that determine what is deemed safe for us to eat but still contradict a vibrant bill of health, we can make the powerful decision to not purchase those products.

When we choose to buy local, organic, plant-based, we inevitably force the food industry to adjust to our demands.

Legislation like the DARK Act shows us that there is no ballot to vote for healthy foods. What we really vote with is our dollars and how we choose to spend them. When we support nutritional and hygiene products that are designed for bottom lines and not for natural health, we support the corrupt system that says it's okay to spray our foods with pesticides, replace standard organic foods with genetically modified foodstuffs, and put chemicals that increase the shelf life of products but reduce human lifespan. I see a lot of people going green using less water and electricity, paper instead of plastic, or switching out their gas guzzler for a Prius, but totally disregard what they're eating and the hygienic products they use.

The Problem with Personal Hygiene Products

Let me first start with hygienic products. Many people have a fear of being condemned to a life of prescription medication. To some degree, this is a healthy fear, according to a 2016 study conducted by John Hopkins University School of Medicine published in *The BMJ* that reported medical error is the third leading cause of death in the U.S., accounting for roughly 10% of all deaths. And when I say 'medical error,' in most cases, these medications were properly prescribed and administered.

So while our apprehension about the pharmaceutical industry and its products is warranted, we seem to overlook hygiene products and deem them as safe and harmless, when in most cases they are quite the opposite. Every time you brush your teeth, roll on deodorant, apply makeup, moisturize your skin with lotion, or use any other hygiene product, you are consuming that product. What most consumers don't know is that the long and complicated list of ingredients on the label is one of the greatest contributors to your

decline in health. If I were able to share with you everything I know

about chemistry, and you then took a look at the average label, you

would have a firm understanding of just how dangerous those

products are and what all those chemical names mean. We consume

these products on a daily basis fresh out of bed and often several

times a day all over our skin, on the scalps of our heads, and inside

our mouths. These daily doses of chemicals go undetected, but their

impact is far from unnoticeable to the educated eye.

Many of the ingredients in beauty products today are actually

pretty ugly. It's impossible for me to educate you on the 80,000-plus

ingredients used in personal care products. However, they contain

industrial chemicals that range from reproductive toxins,

carcinogens, hormone disruptors, pesticides, and heavy metals.

Let's just evaluate a typical deodorant, as an example. If you

were to look at the anatomy of a woman's breast in connection with

the lymphatic system under the armpit, you would be able to see

how intimately connected the two are. The lymph nodes under the

armpit are the first place breast cancer is likely to spread. Lymph

nodes are located primarily in the folds of the body, such as behind the knee, groin, and the armpit. These are areas we sweat the most in order to remove toxins and infections that are collected by the lymphatic channels and excreted out of the lymph nodes. Using anti-perspiration deodorants reduces perspiration and thus causes toxins to build up, which creates the perfect environment for cancer to thrive.

In addition, most deodorants contain cancer-causing paraben chemicals that mimic estrogen activity. Studies have shown that in 99% of breast cancer patients, paraben esters were found.

Start reading the ingredient labels on your products. You can spot these chemicals often listed as methyl, ethyl, propyl, or butylparaben. These same chemicals are also present in shampoos, conditioners, shaving gels, toothpaste, lotions, makeup, and food additives.

This provides a clearer picture of how we unknowingly give ourselves daily doses of cancer.

It's supremely important to remember that anything we apply to our skin is absorbed through our pores and rapidly passed into our bloodstream. Applying chemicals to your skin is in many ways more dangerous than ingesting them. Because via oral administration, there are enzymes in both our mouth and stomach that aid in the metabolism and elimination of these chemicals. Most women are using ten or more beauty products daily, and often they are expired.

The harmful combination of all of the chemicals from the various products has a tremendous impact on your long-term health. It has been estimated that women who wear make-up on a daily basis absorb roughly five pounds of chemicals into their bodies annually. While there is no man, including myself, who wouldn't encourage women to be glamorous and beautiful, I want to implore women to take an organic approach through plant-based nutrition, fitness, and selecting natural products that are consistent with human biology.

Beauty products are a largely unregulated industry, so even labels are difficult to trust; so find a strong brand that stands by its products' ingredients. Below is a list of the Dirty Dozen chemicals for you to look out for. My rule of thumb is, if it has more than five ingredients (especially ingredients having scientific-sounding names), no matter how fancy it looks, it's trash, and you should leave it on the shelf.

The Dirty Dozen Chemicals

1. Parabens

Used in a variety of cosmetics as preservatives. Suspected endocrine disrupters and may interfere with male reproductive functions.

2. Polyethylene glycol (PEG) compounds

Used in many cosmetic cream bases. Can be contaminated with 1,4-dioxane, which may cause cancer. Also related to the chemical propylene glycol and other ingredients with the letters 'eth' (e.g., polyethylene glycol).

3. Butylated hydroxyanisole (BHA)

Most often found in exfoliants, perfumes, moisturizers, and makeup as preservatives. BHA is a suspected endocrine disruptor and carcinogen. In animal studies, BHA has also been shown to increase the risk of stomach cancers, liver damage, thyroid hormone imbalances, and abnormal reproductive development.

4. Coal tar dyes

Coal tar is a byproduct of coal processing. According to the International Agency for Research on Cancer, it is a known human carcinogen. It has been banned in the European Union. It can be commonly found in hair dyes and products listed for dandruff and psoriasis. It's commonly listed on the packaging as p-phenylenediamine in hair dyes. In other products, it can be identified as 'CI' followed by five digits. It may also be listed as 'FD&C Blue No. 1' or 'Blue 1.' In addition to its harmful carcinogenic potential, it may be contaminated with heavy metals toxins.

5. Diethanolamine (DEA)

Closely related to the chemicals TEA and MEA, DEA can react in the body to form nitrosamines, which have the potential to be carcinogenic. It is most often used as an emulsifier and foaming agent in soaps, shampoos, and moisturizers.

6. Phthalates

Phthalates are solvents commonly found in cosmetic products and deodorants. They are also used to make plastics soft and flexible. They can also be used as a plasticizer in some nail care products. These chemicals are suspected in organ damage, endocrine disruption, carcinogenic activity, and reproductive toxicity. When reading labels, look for the abbreviations DEP, DEHP, DBP, DMP, or BzBP to help identify these toxins.

7. Formaldehyde

Despite its presence in the United States, formaldehyde has been banned in the European Union. You will find it listed as diazolidinyl urea, imidazolidinyl urea, DMDM hydantoin, methenamine, and quarternium-15. Most commonly found in hair dyes, fake eyelash adhesives, hair extension glues, and nail products. Has been linked to cancer.

8. Fragrance (Parfum)

Parfum ingredients can often trigger headaches, dizziness, allergies, and asthma. This chemical can be found in soaps, perfumes, shampoos, and even products listed as 'unscented.' Some linked to cancer and neurotoxicity.

9. Mineral oil

A by-product of petroleum often found in hair products to add shine and moisture. Commonly found in baby oils, lipsticks, styling gels, and moisturizers. Petroleum products are often contaminated with polycyclic aromatic hydrocarbons, which are linked to cancer.

10. Paraphenylenediamine (PPD)

PPD is a chemical substance commonly found in permanent hair color and other dyes. PPD can cause reactions ranging from mild skin irritation to more severe allergic contact dermatitis—a form of skin inflammation and irritation commonly referred to as eczema.

11. Talc

Talc has been linked to ovarian cancer. It is commonly found in talcum powders, baby powders, foaming cosmetics, genital deodorants, and bubble bath.

12. Triclosan

Commonly found in antibacterial soaps, hand sanitizers, toothpaste, and antiperspirants. May contribute to antibiotic resistance and has been associated with being an endocrine disruptor.

There are so many more chemicals that didn't make the list but are equally dangerous: aluminum, lead, mercury, hydroquinone, toluene, and sodium lauryl sulfate.

We need to stop counting calories and start counting the chemicals on the label. There are over 10,000 chemicals that are allowed in the American food supply and personal care products that are banned in the EU and countries like Japan. So you can easily see why it's tremendously important to go green not only with your food choices but your hygiene and cosmetic products as well.

Damage to Our Soil and Our Food Chain

The way food is grown today has completely ruined the nutritional quality of much of our soil. Mono-cropping, ammonium nitrate fertilizers, chemical pesticides, and the influx of genetically modified foods have raped our once fertile soils of nutrition.

Good soil requires over fifty minerals and nutrients (calcium, zinc, potassium, manganese, phosphorous, nitrogen, sulfur, etc.). Today much of our soil is primarily composed of just nitrogen, phosphorous, and potassium. As demineralization continues to increase, disease rates rise in the same parallel fashion. In the

documentary *Food Matters*, Charlotte Gershon of the Gershon
Institute couldn't have stated it better: "When the soil is deficient,
the plant is deficient, and so insects attack and pesticides are used."
It's a vicious inorganic cycle that is at the forefront of our health
disparity.

Now consider that most of the produce that is eaten is
canned, boxed, and frozen, and then we add insult to injury by
overcooking it. Studies have shown that even when you lightly
prepare your food by steaming it, you kill crucial enzymes. In the
1930s, a Swiss doctor named Dr. Kouchakoff proved through
numerous studies that a diet consisting of greater than 51% cooked
foods was detrimental to your health, and our immune system
reacted as if overly cooked foods were a foreign invader. These
studies also showed that a diet that consisted of less than 51%
cooked foods did not produce digestive leukocytosis. This is why it
is paramount that we eat more raw foods to be properly nourished,
build immunity, and prevent disease.

In my opinion, it's ridiculous to be charged more for organic
food when it has fewer chemicals and no genetic altering. It's like
ordering a hamburger with no cheese or burger and getting charged

extra. But our entire food system in America is in so much disarray

we accept this type of behavior in exchange for nutritionally poor

foods with cheap prices.

The mechanization of farming has ruined the quality of foods

we eat. Dr. Rebecca Dunnings of the Kenan Institute for Ethics

conducted research on the effects of genetic engineering and the

pesticide glyphosate on mineral content in the mid-1990s. Her work

showed that in order to get the same amount of iron you would have

gotten from an apple in 1950, it would require you to eat 26 apples

in 1998. This explains why food today doesn't taste nearly as good

as it once did, so the food industry adulterates it with chemical

sugars and additives to compensate its tasteless remix of nature.

It's Time You Get Some Vegucation!

The modern foods we eat today have had their nutrients

removed through a refining process, and then they are laced with

inorganic vitamins and minerals that could never replace those in

whole foods. In addition, it seems people are under the assumption

that a multivitamin (whether plant-based or synthetic) is capable of

being the 'magic pill' to all of this madness. Well, I'm here to vegucate you. There is no 'magic pill.' Stop believing there is or will be. A plant-based, whole foods lifestyle is the standalone solution to our health crisis. So buy produce that is in season, local, and organic as much as possible.

The fiber in plant-based whole foods can make transitioning away from the SAD diet uncomfortable because you'll have to chew your food more than you ever have compared to the soft mushy foods you're used to, and initially, you probably won't have enough stomach acid to digest these foods in their entirety. This will initially cause some gas and bloating as the bacteria in your digestive system begin to adjust to your new way of living. Don't worry; your body will adjust, and you'll have a new microbiome to thank yourself for. Begin by implementing green smoothies and juices every morning. Green smoothies aren't just a meal replacement; they can be an actual meal that fills you up because of the fiber and nutritional content that satiates you.

The key word is 'green' smoothie, not 'fruit' smoothie. The foundation of your smoothies should be green leafy vegetables along with herbs like cilantro, parsley, and basil. According to the Hippocrates Health Institute, a deeper green pigment indicates the richness of the chlorophyll present in the plant, which directly corresponds to a more abundant health-building quality. Chlorophyll aids in healing wounds, inflammation, normalizing blood clotting, digestive health, deodorizing, detoxification, hormonal balance, and binds up toxic heavy metals to hamper their absorption. Chlorophyll is to plants what blood is to humans and much more. The structure of chlorophyll parallels the hemoglobin molecule present in both humans and animals. Hemoglobin can be found in our red blood cells and is responsible for carrying oxygen from our lungs to organs and tissues. When we compare a hemoglobin and chlorophyll molecule side by side, the only difference is at the center of the porphyrin ring, where hemoglobin retains an iron atom and chlorophyll retains a magnesium atom. This is why increasing the chlorophyll content in your diet by way of green smoothies is unequivocally one of the greatest biohacks you can implement for your own well-being.

Many of the blood-building components required for a healthy blood supply can found in many of the chlorophyll-rich foods that you'll be tossing into your blender.

Making Your Green Smoothies

Especially for those who've mostly consumed a SAD diet, in the beginning, you will find the transition will be harsh on your chewing muscles, taste buds, and even your stomach. The digestive discomfort is the cleansing effect of chlorophyll sweeping through your body, ridding itself of years of pollution. You've been starved of solar power in the form of chlorophyll for far too long, but once the deficit is replenished, you'll find yourself with a renewed set of taste buds, a 20/20-like mental clarity, and a slimmer waistline by way of the appetite suppressive effects of chlorophyll.

The other huge plus with green smoothies that you won't receive from a SAD diet is, you get a massive amount of fiber, which blunts the glycemic spike while cleansing and detoxing your colon.

When making your smoothies, make sure that the proportions of greens to fruits is about 70% greens to 30% fruits. Of course, it's okay to make a tasty strawberry banana smoothie at times, but be sure to make the 70/30 split your foundation.

Another vital gem is to ensure that you are constantly rotating your greens and herbs in your smoothies. This is important because each green has different vitamins, minerals, trace elements, and phytonutrients. Maintaining a green variety ensures you will get the full spectrum of nutrients that are available and also prevents you from accumulating certain compounds like oxalic acid, which is present in spinach and can combine with calcium from your bones, leading to kidney stones and osteoporosis.

Also add superfoods, seeds, and sea vegetables to keep diversity in your nutritional deposits.

If you like creamy smoothies, you can use bananas, avocados, flax or chia seeds, coconut meat, or nut butters. The key to getting that restaurant-like quality is the blender, so I would recommend investing in a high-quality appliance. The keyword is 'investing,' because you can either pay Big Pharma or the farmer—the choice is yours!

Lastly, don't be concerned about the sugar content from fruit. These are natural sugars combined with fiber, which blunts the glycemic spike that would normally occur with processed and refined foods. Nature's already figured out the solution; just fall into alignment, and your body will handle the rest. As long as the fruits are seasonal and not hybrids, you shouldn't be worried, especially if you're avoiding added sugars.

PLANT-BASED STARTER KIT

RECLAIM
YOUR HEALTH

Dr. Bobby Price

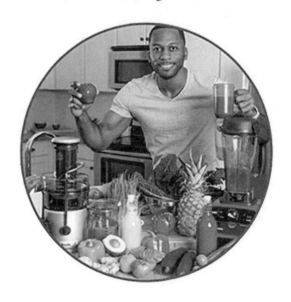

Welcome Letter

Greetings!

I'm Dr. Bobby Price, author
of Vegucation Over Medication,
and your Plant-based Pharmacist
and Nutritionist.

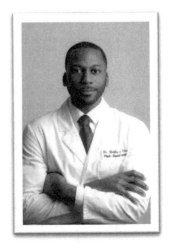

After personally
experiencing the healing powers of
a plant-based lifestyle sevens years
ago I was inspired to adopt a more
holistic approach to healing. Since that time I've traveled the world
studying with herbalists, shamans, and spiritual gurus learning the
magical art of healing the mind, body, and soul. In my upcoming
book **"Vegucation Over Medication,"** I talked about the unknown
dangers in modern foods and medicines, and how a plant-based
lifestyle is capable of preventing and reversing disease. Stay tuned
for its release APRIL 2018!

My hope is to inspire and empower you with holistic
teachings that help you **RECLAIM YOUR HEALTH**.

My philosophy on wellness is an integrative approach that focuses not just on the body, but the mind and soul as well during the healing process. I'll show you easy and tasteful ways to incorporate organic plant-based food in your diet. But I will also be teaching you about natural remedies, herbal medicine, and ancient healing techniques like meditation and yoga.

In this Holistic ReEngineering Jump Starter Kit, I'll explain why diets don't work and this lifestyle does. You'll also learn how the toxic nature of modern foods, drugs, thinking, television, and relationships can all be cleansed by being Holistically ReEngineered by nature.

While this is just a starter kit, it is absolutely essential and foundational to you making a successful transition to a healthy and balanced lifestyle. For more awesome information like this, follow me on Instagram @doctorholistic, Facebook @drbobbyprice, or email me at info@drbobbyprice.com. You can also ask me about my herbal Parasite Candida cleanse for the digestive system which I highly recommend. Remember all disease begins in the gut.

P.S. This is a judgment free love zone. So I encourage you to move at your own pace and embrace the journey. If it all seems like too much at once just embrace what resonates with you now and add

more layers as your comfort level grows.

DR. BOBBY PRICE

Beyond all I wish you prosperity in your mind, body, and soul.

7 MAJOR KEYS FOR A SEAMLESS TRANSITION TO A PLANT-BASED LIFESTYLE

1. Decide how you will transition. Omnivore to Vegetarian then Plant-based Vegan, Vegetarian then Plant-based Vegan, or Cold Turkey Vegan. The choice is yours, but you should definitely decide because as they say those without a plan, plan to fail. Although there is no winning or losing in transitioning your lifestyle you do want to accomplish what you set out to do.

2. Preparation is a MAJOR KEY! Most people I've worked with often have great initial experiences with transitioning to a plant-based vegan lifestyle, but lack of preparation has been the most consistent downfall. Eventually after all the excitement and newness of life without animal-based products wears off most are stuck trying to figure out what to eat, feel like their starving themselves when there's a lack of healthy options, and end up over spending on eating out and grocery shopping. So it's key to be prepared by having a list of go to restaurants that support your lifestyle in your local

area, a list of great go to recipes for quick meals, and shopping at grocery stores for meals and quick healthy snacks not groceries. When you shop for meals and snacks you avoid getting home to bags of random items that can't be assembled into something you want to eat.

3. Add Before You Subtract. This means before you go cold turkey try a few vegan restaurants locally and a few recipes at home. Begin switching up your grocery list to more plant-based foods by trying meat alternatives, healthier grains lie quinoa, superfoods, and drinking only natural spring water. Adding more plant-based foods while gradually transitioning animal products out of your pantry allows you the time you need to transition seamlessly.

4. Walk in silence. There's absolutely no need for you to make a huge announcement with your family or friends, or on social media that you've decided to embrace a healthier lifestyle of nutrition. You can be certain that if you do people you haven't spoken to in years will come out of nowhere pressuring you to defend your healthy decision. Isn't it

funny, that as soon as you decide to eat healthier, everyone all of sudden becomes a nutritionist? Here's a great tip. Don't take nutrition advice from someone who eats 5 slices of bacon every morning even though the World Health Organization has classified bacon and meats like it level one carcinogens. Allow yourself the space to grow in your own decision and only tell those who support you making a healthier choice for you and the environment.

5. Get yourself a Vegucation! It highly important with any major decision to start with WHY? When you know your why your decision takes on purpose, its not about a label or following the trend. Learn about the benefits of embracing a plant-based vegan lifestyle. Watch inspirational and educational documentaries like Earthlings, Food Inc., Eating You Alive, Forks Over Knives, and Food Matters. This will help give you a WHY and answer many of the pressing questions that probably delayed you from making the transition to begin with.

6. Don't get stuck in transition. The demand for vegan and vegetarian food skyrocketed up 987% in 2017. With this exponential demand, many plant-based food companies are using some of the same techniques to process plant-based foods to compete with our old omnivorous taste buds. Although, these foods are delicious and great for transitioning to a plant-based vegan diet they are not whole foods. Which means you can survive eating them, but cannot thrive eating anything that has been isolated and processed. This is one of the major reasons why it's very common to see someone who is either vegan or vegetarian for years and they may still be overweight and unhealthy. So its ok to eat these foods sparingly and during your transition, but the focus is health and wellbeing.

7. Cleanse and detox. It shouldn't be any surprise to anyone that for the majority of people eating whole fruits, vegetables, seeds, and nuts don't satisfy our taste buds initially. After decades of eating adulterated versions of food, the taste of natural whole foods might be a foreign concept. In addition, processed foods lack the vitality, fiber,

and micronutrients that nourish our digestive tracts so it lays the ground for nasty critters to flourish like parasites and candida. This is why I highly recommend beginning your transition with an herbal cleanse that will silence the critters and ultimately silence the phantom cravings your have for salt, sugar, and fat. Also doing an herbal cleanse versus your conventional variety nourishes the tissues and detoxes the body of harmful chemicals stored in the body's fat tissues. Once you remove the toxins from fat the pounds will start melting away like vegan butter!

Plant-based Meat Replacements

- Mushrooms
- Jackfruit
- Nut meat
- Chickpea
- Black beans
- Lentils
- Eggplant
- Cauliflower

Plant-based Seed and Nut Milks

- Flaxseed milk
- Coconut milk
- Almond milk

Plant-based Cheese Replacements

- Cashew based
- Pine nut based
- Almonds
- Nutritional yeast (sparingly)

*There are many prepackaged version of cheese you can easily purchase at your local health food store. But I highly recommend you do this sparingly and as an alternative make your own in a high powered food processor. I'll add a plant-based cheese recipe for you to try at home.

Plant-based Egg Replacements

- Flaxseed Meal (1 tbsp + 3 tbsp water)
- Chia Seeds (1 tbsp + 3 tbsp water)
- Banana (1/4 cup)
- Pumpkin + Sweet Potato (1/4 cup)
- Avocado (1/4 cup)

Plant-based Suggested Cooking Oils

- Avocado oil
- Hempseed oil
- Grapeseed oil
- Sesame oil
- Coconut oil (do not cook with this oil)
- Olive oil (do not cook with this oil)

PLANT BASED SHOPPING LIST

Vegetables

Kale	Onion
Cucumbers	Zucchini
Olives	Squash
Avocado	Tomato (cherry & plum only)
Turnip greens	Okra
All lettuce (except iceberg)	Watercress
Green banana	Bell peppers
Bok Choy	Garbanzo beans/Chickpeas
Mushrooms (not shitake)	Spinach (in moderation)
Romaine lettuce	

Fruits

Mangoes	Berries
Dates	Prunes
Grapes	Pears
Peaches	Cherries
Apples (organic)	Peaches
Prickly Pear	Banana (small or midsized)
Limes	Plums
Cantaloupe	Melons
Raisins	

*All fruits must be seeded

Grains

Quinoa	Amaranth
Fonio	Kamut
Spelt	Amaranth
Wild rice	Teff

Spices

Pink Himalayan Sea Salt
Cayenne pepper
Parsley
Basil
Dill
Bay leaf

Oregano
Onion powder
Cilantro
Clove
Thyme
Turmeric

Nuts & Seeds

Walnuts
Almonds
Hemp seeds
Sesame seeds (raw)

Tahini
Brazilian nuts
Pecans
Flaxseed

*Be sure to presoak your almonds before consuming

Sweeteners

Pure agave syrup (cactus)   Dates

Oils

Hempseed oil
Sesame oil
Coconut oil (do not cook)

Avocado oil
Grapeseed oil
Olive oil (do not cook)

Beverages

Natural Spring water (directly from the source)
Coconut water (directly from the coconut)

*You can infuse the spring water with cucumber, mint, key limes, or oranges.

Herbs and Superfoods

Burdock	Anise
Valerian	Allspice
Ginger root	Chamomile
Sea moss (powder and gel)	Fennel
Chlorella	Turmeric root
Bladderwrack	Elderberry
Hemp (powder or seed)	Chamomile
Linden	

Its important to note this is the strict guideline for foods to purchase when at the local farmer's market or grocery store. You'll find there are a few things in my recipes that are not on the list. Those are things I encourage you to eat very sparingly. Stick to the shopping list as much as possible. And drink a green Juice or Smoothie every morning for breakfast for the best results. Doing every morning is what provides the cleansing you need for healing and health

This is my dirty dozen list to always buy organic and my clean 15 that you can buy conventional at the grocery store.

Dirty Dozen +2	Clean 15
1. Apples	1. Onions
2. Blueberries	2. Avocado
3. Walnuts	3. Pineapples
4. Cucumbers	4. Mango
5. Grapes	5. Sweet Peas
6. Kale	6. Eggplant
7. Peaches	7. Chickpeas
8. Potatoes	8. Asparagus
9. Papaya (esp. from Hawaii)	9. Kiwi
10. Strawberries	10. Cabbage
11. Sweet bell peppers	11. Melons (seeded)
12. Tomatoes	12. Soursop
	13. Quinoa
+ Corn	14. Zucchini
+ All soy products	15. Coconuts

VEGAN FOOD RECIPES (BONUS!)

Great Guacamole

- 2 avocados
- 1 bunch of cilantro
- $1/4$ of a medium sized red onion
- $1/2$ of a lime squeezed (key lime)
- Black Olives
- Cherry tomatoes
- Cayenne Pepper
- Himalayan Pink Salt
- Stone Ground Black Pepper

*1/2 Squeezed Mandarin Orange (optional)

Black bean Mushroom Burgers

- 1 cup of cooked quinoa
- 1 & 1/3 cups canned black beans mashed
- 1 tbsp. olive oil for frying
- 7 medium sized mushrooms finely chopped
- 2 tsp of ground cumin
- 2 tbsp. of Sriracha
- $1/4$ red onion finely chopped
- 2 garlic gloves finely minced
- 1&1/2-2 cups of bread crumbs
- 1 tbsp. of ground chia seed or flaxseed
- 2 tbsp. of nutritional yeast
- 2&1/2 tbsp. of Braggs Liquid Aminos
- Squeeze lemon juice
- 3 tbsp. of water
- Season with Himalayan pink salt and cracked black pepper

*Mix all ingredients in one container and refrigerate for an hour before making patties and cooking. Serve with lettuce, tomato, and sliced avocado

Curried Chickpea Salad

- 3 cups cooked or 2 (15 oz.) cans of chickpeas (garbanzo beans) drained and rinsed
- 1 cup of organic carrots
- 1 cups of scallions/green onions diced
- 1/2 cup of raisins or chopped dates
- 1/2 a cup of raw cashews
- 1/2 to 2/3 cups of tahini or hummus
- juice of 1 lemon
- 1 tablespoon of curry powder
- 3/4 teaspoon of garlic powder
- Himalayan Pink salt and cracked pepper to taste

Vegan Cheese Wiz

- 4 c red jacket potatoes, chopped
- 1 $^1/_2$ c fresh carrots, diced large
- $^1/_2$ c water
- $^1/_3$ extra virgin olive oil
- $^1/_2$ c nutritional yeast
- 1 tbsp. lemon juice
- 1 tsp onion powder
- 1 tsp garlic powder
- 1 tsp parsley
- 1/2 tsp all spice seasoning
- Salt/Pepper to taste

Instructions

1. Steam or boil the potatoes and carrots until tender.
2. Now place everything into a blender and run until smooth and creamy.
3. Add to macaroni, nachos, or lasagna

Avocado Tahini Dressing

- 1 avocado
- ½ of a medium sized green pepper
- 2 tbsp. of tahini
- 1 tbsp. of pure agave nectar
- pinch of Himalayan seal salt
- 1 tsp of coconut vinegar

Thank You!

As our journey together in this book comes to an end, I hope that your plant-based journey towards good health and happiness has just begun. Let me first say how proud of you I am for embracing one of the greatest acts of self-love there is: improving your own health. In my opinion, health is the greatest form of wealth. With it, anything is possible; without it, nothing is. As a bonus, I created a plant-based starter kit to help make your transition a little more seamless. Enjoy it and apply it, and it will surely help you and your loved ones reclaim their health!